Nurse Executive Study Guide 2023-2024

ANCC Review + 450 Test Questions and Detailed Answer Explanations for Certification (Includes 3 Full-Length Exams)

Printed in the United States of America

Table of Contents

Chapter 1: What the Nurse Executive Exam Entails

The Nurse Executive Exam evaluates whether a nurse is competent enough to receive the NE-BC credentials, awarded by the American Nurses Credentialing Center (ANCC) Nurse Executive Board.

NE-BC stands for "Nurse Executive-Board Certified." The credentials assure employers that a certified nurse is sufficiently knowledgeable and skilled in clinical matters to be able to handle the day-to-day operations of a medical institution.

The NE-BC certification is accredited by the National Commission for Certifying Agencies and the Accreditation Board for Specialty Nursing Certification. The NE-BC certification is valid for five years. Then it must be renewed.

Requirements for Taking the NE Exam

It is important to keep in mind that there are conditions one needs to fulfill in order to be allowed to take the exam. By the time you seek certification as a nurse executive, you should already have qualified as a registered nurse (RN). After being certified as a NE-BC, your hands-on skills as an RN will help you fulfill your administrative duties while in a managerial position at a health-care facility. The RN license must be recognized in the state within which the candidate is seeking certification as a NE-BC.

Registered nurses normally support physicians with duties that include performing medical exams and dispensing medications, as well as operating medical equipment.

Certified nurse executives oversee the daily tasks at a medical facility, along with operations of a long-term nature like budget management. Other long-term tasks entrusted to nurse executives include the deployment of personnel and valuable assets and playing a leadership role at the hospital level. Nurse executives are considered competent enough to run medical centers and nursing homes, as well as community-based clinics and any other health-care organization.

Some large health institutions have nurse executives who manage respective health units, so that a pediatric unit, for example, is supervised by one nurse executive. It is important to note that the nurse executives entrusted with overseeing the affairs of a big hospital are at a higher level than those nurse executives who are newly certified.

Prerequisites to Becoming a NE-BC

Before becoming a NE-BC, you need to be an RN.

You must have a high school diploma or a GED. With that certification you can apply to any of the nursing programs or medical colleges in the country. Note that you stand a better chance of being accepted into a program if you have performed particularly well in biology and chemistry, as well as math. Having psychology as one of your disciplines could also improve your chances.

Some high school graduates choose to study courses that are considered part of pre-nursing coursework, which include anatomy, psychology, physiology and microbiology, as well as subjects like sociology, statistics and others.

Although being a licensed RN is sufficient qualification for someone intending to take the nurse executive exam, some people also go on to get a master of science in nursing (MSN), which opens up new career paths. Others take business programs and healthcare-related administration courses.

Professional Requirements for a NE-BC

Another requirement for anyone preparing to be certified as a NE-BC is that they must have experience working in an administrative or supervisory capacity for at least two of the last three years, generally in middle-level management. In addition, all candidates except those with an MSN need to have covered 30 hours of continuing education within the area of nursing administration.

There is also special consideration given to RNs who have been working as instructors, tutors or consultants in the field of nursing administration.

Difference between NE-BC & NEA-BC

It is important to know there is a distinction between NE-BC and NEA-BC, although both are certifications for nurse executives. The former has already been discussed in the book, while the latter, NEA-BC, stands for Nurse Executive Advanced-Board Certified. Both courses are administered by the ANCC.

The major difference between the two professional certifications is that the level of education to qualify for an NEA-BC certification is higher than what is required for the NE-BC.

Nurse Executive Exam Structure

The nurse executive exam is computer-based, and it comprises 150 questions, twenty-five of which are not scored. The questions are multiple-choice, with each having four answer choices, of which only one is correct.

Candidates should pay equal attention to all the questions, as the twenty-five questions which are not scored are not marked.

The time provided for the entire exam is three and a half hours.

Any candidate whose score is 350 and over is considered to have passed the exam, and therefore is qualified for the NE-BC certification. The maximum a candidate can score on the exam is 500.

Areas of Study

The questions in the NE-BC exam are derived from four major areas of study: **Human Resource Management (31%), Quality and Safety (21%), Business Management (14%) and Health Care Delivery (34%)**. Each section is divided into knowledge and skills on the ANCC exam outline. Each area also has subtopics that are important to study.

The following chapters contain the information you need to prepare for all four major test sections. Many of the questions that are included in the practice tests at the end of the book have answers that can be found in these chapters.

Chapter 2: Human Resource Management – Knowledge

One of the major areas of study for aspiring nurse executives comprises the human resources found in health organizations, where nurse executives are likely to be employed after certification.

A nurse executive's position in an organization is an administrative one, and therefore nurse executives must know a great deal about human resources.

The dominant factor in a health-care institution is the workforce that renders care to patients at varying levels. In order for an institution to run efficiently and for service delivery to be up to par, relevant laws and regulations must be followed, and the nurse executive has to ensure that happens.

That is why it is important that nurse executives be well versed in federal laws and other laws that guide the provision of health care in the US.

The Laws at Federal & State Level

It is up to the nurse executive to ensure that any federal or state laws relating to the running of health institutions are adhered to.

The Family & Medical Leave Act

The Family & Medical Leave Act (FMLA) was enacted in 1993, and it stipulates that any organization with a workforce of fifty employees should provide for unpaid absences or leave without jeopardizing employees' jobs.

Conditions for Unpaid Absence

An employee's job is protected for twelve weeks within a period of one year, and acceptable reasons for granting such leave include medical issues and family matters. If the leave is sought on medical grounds, the employee must not be able to execute his/her normal duties properly. Leave sought on the basis of family grounds includes caring for an infant, caring for a spouse who is indisposed or caring for a child or parent.

For employees to qualify for such unpaid leave, they must be employed on either a full-time or part-time basis. Also, they must have worked at the institution for over 1,250 hours in the preceding year.

An employee entitled to such leave will continue to receive work benefits, including insurance coverage. If, when the employee returns to work, his/her employer wants to give the employee a position different from the one previously held, the new position must come with a salary, benefits and responsibilities commensurate with the previous job the person held.

Special Concession for Service Members

If an employee is applying for unpaid leave for the sake of taking care of a spouse who is a service member, the leave and its concurrent benefits may be extended to twenty-six weeks within the stipulated twelve-month duration. This extended leave of absence should also be granted if the reason for applying for it is to care for a child or service member.

The Americans with Disabilities Act

The Americans with Disabilities Act (ADA) ensures the civil rights of any American with a disability of any kind are respected, and that includes being given an equal chance at employment. It is important to note that the people protected by this act include those whose impairment is of a mental nature.

Chronic Ailments Considered Under the ADA

Although the ADA is meant to protect people with disabilities, these do not have to be obvious ones like being blind; they include conditions like arthritis, seizures, cardiovascular problems and disorders of a respiratory nature.

Since communities are also obligated to observe the ADA, they are expected to provide transport services that are convenient for people with disabilities, including providing wheelchairs. By extension, health institutions should provide the same, as they are also a community. Health facilities must ensure they are accessible to people with disabilities by installing elevators and ramps.

Institutions should also ensure they have modes of communication convenient for people with disabilities, like devices that the hearing and vision impaired can use.

Although nurse executives should be conversant with the stipulations of the ADA, they should also take note that there are old structures that are limited in how far they can go to fulfill the law's requirements. However, on the whole, the nurse executive should see to it that the stipulations of the ADA are adhered to, and where that has not happened, make the necessary recommendations.

The Fair Labor Standards Act

The Fair Labor Standards Act (FLSA) stipulates what the minimum remuneration should be for employees, the rate of overtime, records to be maintained and what constitutes child labor. The minimum wage set by the federal government in 2009 was $7.25 per hour, and overtime was paid at the rate of one and a half times the normal rate. Overtime begins counting after forty working hours in a week.

When the State Minimum is Higher than the Federal Minimum Wage

It is important to note that a state can legislate to have its minimum wage be higher than that of the federal minimum wage, and nurse executives should learn the laws in their respective states, so as to ensure their institutions adhere accordingly. When state and federal laws on wages vary, employees are entitled to the higher salary.

In those businesses where employees earn over $30 per month in the form of tips, the law demands that they be paid that money directly, and the rate should reflect a minimum hourly rate of $2.13.

Authority to Pay Below Minimum Wage

There are instances where the law permits employers to pay certain employees' wages below the federal minimum wage. Among those affected by this exemption from the law are students and people with disabilities that significantly affect their productivity. As for hospitals, they sometimes have partial exemptions regarding overtime.

Partial Exemption for Hospitals

An example of a partial exemption for a hospital is where employees in a given unit have a fourteen-week schedule rather than the usual seven-day week. While this is acceptable under the law because of the health sector's unique circumstances, the employees are entitled to overtime for any hours they work after eight hours of any day. Alternatively, for every fourteen-day session, employees are entitled to overtime for all shifts worked beyond eighty hours.

National Labor Relations Act

The National Labor Relations Act was enacted in 1935 to ensure that employees would have the right for collective bargaining and prevent specific companies from exploiting their workers through questionable management procedures.

Wage & Hour Laws

While some of these laws may not seem to affect hospitals and other health institutions, nurse executives need to be conversant with them, because the institutions in which they work relate to other organizations as well. As such, hospital administrators need to ensure their institutions treat those stakeholders, including suppliers, according to the law.

FLSA and FMLA, already explained, fall under this category of wage and hour laws. Other legislation under this category includes the Davis-Bacon Act; the Walsh-Healy Public Contracts Act; Contract Work Hours & Safety Standards Act; McNamara-O'Hara Service Contract Act and the Federal Wage Garnishment Law.

The Davis-Bacon Act

This act stipulates that any contractor or subcontractor handling any public works project should be compensated at the prevailing wage rate.

The Walsh-Healy Public Contracts Act

This act sets the rate for overtime wages and also establishes the minimum wages an employee can legally receive if working under a government contract whose worth exceeds $10,000, manufacturing goods or equipment or supplying them.

Contract Work Hours & Safety Standards Act

This act stipulates that any contractor or subcontractor handling a federal contract whose worth exceeds $100,000 must pay overtime at the rate of one and a half times per hour, for every hour over forty hours a week.

This same act prohibits employers from exposing their employees to conditions that are unsanitary or unsafe.

McNamara-O'Hara Service Contract Act

According to this act, any contractor or subcontractor handling a contract worth more than $2,500 should pay employees the wages prevailing at the time. If the contract's worth is below $2,500, then employees should be paid the minimum wage, if not better.

Federal Wage Garnishment Law

This law protects employees with regard to garnishment because it limits the extent, in monetary terms, to which anyone can garnish an employee's wages. Employers are prohibited from terminating employees on account of wage garnishment.

Laws on Equal Employment

There are a number of laws that have been enacted over the years for the purpose of ensuring the US offers equal employment opportunities to everyone.

The EEOC

The Equal Employment Opportunity Commission (EEOC) is responsible for ensuring that employers do not discriminate against employees. The organizations under the watch of the EEOC must have fifteen employees or more, but in matters relating to age discrimination, the employees must be at least twenty in number. Other organizations under the purview of the EEOC are labor unions and employment agencies.

The 1964 Civil Rights Act, Title VII

This law operates alongside the Pregnancy Discrimination Act and prohibits employers from discriminating against employees on account of their race, gender, country of origin, religion and/or pregnancy.

The 1991 Civil Rights Act

The sections of this law relevant to the role of nurse executives are sections 102 and 103. These have caused amendments to past laws, and led to trials by jury, resulting in financial compensation and punitive damages.

The 1963 Equal Pay Act

As per this law, employers should pay equal amounts to both male and female employees, as long as they are performing work equally.

The 1967 ADEA

The Age Discrimination in Employment Act (ADEA) is meant mainly to protect employees who are age forty and over.

The 1990 ADA

The Americans with Disabilities Act, which has already been explained in this book, also falls under equal employment laws. This law protects employees under state governments and their agencies, those employed by local authorities, as well as those employed in the private sector.

Candidates with disabilities seeking employment need to be qualified for the available position, and their disabilities should be such that they can be reasonably accommodated by employers.

The 1973 Rehabilitation Act

The sections of this act relevant to the role of a nurse executive are 501 and 505. The implications and operations of these sections are like the ADA's, with the difference being that the targeted employer is the federal government.

The 2008 GINA

The Genetic Information Non-Discrimination Act (GINA) stipulates that employers are forbidden from discriminating against any employee on account of information pertaining to genes. The motivation behind the enactment of this law was that certain people are prone to some genetic ailments, and it was feared that some insurance providers might consider these individuals more risky than other clients and could possibly raise their premiums or reject them.

Occupational Safety & Health Administration

The Occupational Safety & Health Administration (OSHA) oversees policies put in place for the control of infections. OSHA requires safeguards to eliminate situations where employees are exposed to infection. It is also a requirement by the FDA that devices intended for medical use be safe.

As a nurse executive, you need to appreciate that the regulations of the state within which you are working might be more stringent than the ones set by OSHA, and your institution is bound by those regulations.

Important OSHA Elements

Every health institution under OSHA's watch is expected to have a plan in place to reduce the chances of staff being injured. Institutions are expected to always adhere to universally accepted precautions, no matter who they are dealing with.

Hospitals are required to have clear working practices for their staff as a way of minimizing dangers in the workplace. They are required to adopt newer technologies as they enter the market if these have been proven to be safer than older devices.

Proper disposal of sharps is also required under OSHA. Sharps should not be bent, recapped, sheared or broken, and needles and other sharps that have been contaminated should be handled safely and disposed of appropriately. It is also important that nurses and other members of staff receive training pertaining to universally accepted sharps precautions.

Staff members need to understand a health-care facility's plan for control of exposure. In addition, health institutions are expected to ensure staff is immunized against hepatitis B.

Workers' Compensation

Workers' compensation benefits employees who are injured in the course of duty. It is offered in three forms: cash as a substitute for wages not earned during illness or injury, reimbursement of any costs incurred when getting treatment for the injury and benefits for the death of the injured employee paid to next of kin.

Laws governing workers' compensation often vary in different states, and correspondingly, it may be easier to access data pertaining to workers' compensation locally than at the national level. The kind of information you can expect to find relates to how frequent and severe certain kinds of injuries are and the magnitude of costs linked to them.

The reason administrators such as nurse executives may benefit from this data is that it can help in designing appropriate safety measures. It can also be of help when deciding the nature of training employees require with regards to the prevention of accidents and safety in general.

Implication of Workers' Compensation for Employers

Once an employee has received workers' compensation, he/she can no longer hold the employer liable for any other costs. This means that acceptance of the insurance benefits is tantamount to the employee waiving the right to enter into litigation against the employer.

However, there are a few exceptions where an employee who has been compensated through workers' compensation has a right to sue the employer. A good example is when a worker is injured after being assaulted by an employer; the relevant charge is intentional tort.

Another exception is when an employer demands that an employee engage in an activity that requires special protection but does not provide the employee with the right gear; the relevant charge is reckless conduct. Also, an employee who is injured in the course of duty but does not receive workers' compensation can sue.

The employee is then obliged to prove to the courts that the employer was negligent.

The Omnibus Budget Reconciliation Act

The 1987 Omnibus Budget Reconciliation Act (OBRA) encompasses the Nursing Home Reform Amendments (NHRA) of 1990, which address the utilization of health-care facilities by nurses, particularly in those institutions that provide care on a long-term basis.

The NHRA provisions include assessing patients during admission, not only for their physical condition but also for their mental health. This type of examination must be performed annually. Another provision is that these patients be taken care of on a twenty-four-hour basis, with RNs on duty a minimum of a single shift a day.

It is also required that nurse aides regularly attend in-services and that the names of the nurse aides be recorded in the registry of their respective states. These institutions are required to provide rehabilitation services for patients. In addition, the patients must be visited by physicians, their assistants or nurse practitioners every thirty days from the time of their admission, and thereafter, every ninety days.

Another of the provisions stipulates that patients should not face discrimination as far as Medicaid is concerned. They should also be independently monitored for psychopharmacologic medications or drugs, with pharmacists ensuring patients are not at risk of drug-related complications.

Under these provisions, it is mandatory that patients' rights are respected. Surveys should be carried out with a view to assessing the kind of care patients are receiving and what the outcomes are. The law provides for state sanctioning, to ensure regulations put in place for the running of nursing homes are adhered to.

The Older Americans Act

The 1965 Older Americans Act (OAA) is a result of Title III, which was modified through the 2006 amendments. This law provides for enhancement of service access by the elderly and Native Americans. The services covered in this respect go beyond health care to include provision of meals and transportation, home care, home repairs and services of a legal nature.

An example of a program that benefits from funds given, courtesy of the OAA, is Meals on Wheels. The funds set aside to help the elderly are distributed as required through local agencies, which are better placed to understand the needs of individuals in respective localities.

The National Family Caregivers Support Act, which was enacted for the purpose of rendering assistance to people caring for the elderly, falls under the OAA. It is also under the OAA that programs have been established to guard against elder abuse. Certain computer literacy programs for the elderly also fall under the heading of the OAA.

The Ombudsman

OAA provides for ombudsman programs so that a resident in any nursing home can have a safe avenue through which to raise grievances. This provision is an attempt to make sure the services provided in nursing homes meet the standards required by respective states.

The Emergency Medical Treatment & Active Labor Act

The Emergency Medical Treatment & Active Labor Act (EMTALA) was enacted to ensure that any patient brought to an ER is provided with appropriate services irrespective of whether or not the person has medical insurance or has the capacity to pay for the services.

Transfer of Patients from the ER

The law allows patients in the ER to be transferred to a ward within the hospital or a different hospital. Such transfers must only be made after the patient has been stabilized, and if the patient is actively in labor, only after she has delivered both the baby and the placenta.

Any screening of such patients should be done before anyone can begin inquiring into matters of insurance or the patient's capacity to pay the medical bill. By the time a decision is made to transfer a patient from the ER, the medical staff should be confident that a patient's condition is unlikely to be worsened in the course of such a transfer.

The institution receiving a patient from the ER must have the capacity to treat the patient's condition. Per the law, the only time an institution is mandated to transfer a patient from one facility to another is when it does not have the capacity to treat the person because of a lack of specialized resources or skills the patient requires, as exemplified by burn cases.

Labor Issues

Labor issues pertain to the relationship employees have with their employers. Nurse executives, who hold administrative positions, need to understand the regulations and contracts pertaining to this relationship. The most prominent one is the Collective Bargaining Agreement (CBA), which involves remuneration.

The Collective Bargaining Agreement

Employees bargain collectively, mostly through their respective unions. The matters normally addressed in this manner include wages and workplace conditions. Whatever agreements the parties arrive at are put together to form the CBA, which is revised from time to time.

An example of a labor union is the United American Nurses, whose CBA, like those of other unions, is governed by federal law as well as the laws of the respective states.

When discussing a CBA, the employer comes to the table as a team of five to seven people, and the employees are represented by a similar number of individuals.

Bargaining Types

There are three major ways of carrying out labor negotiations: distributive, integrative and mixed. The distributive negotiation entails a process that is competitive, where one side emerges the winner while the other side loses. It is known as "zero-sum; win-lose." When this manner of bargaining is utilized, the parties either end up coming to a compromise, or they are at a stalemate at the end of the negotiations.

The integrative manner of negotiating is collaborative. The two parties bargain as partners, meaning jointly, with the intention of resolving any existing problem to both parties' mutual satisfaction.

The mixed form of negotiation applies tactics from both the distributive and integrative processes.

Negotiating Contracts

Contracts are negotiated between employees and an institution's administration. Preparing for contract negotiations involves reviewing notes and reports that were recorded during the most recent negotiations; collection of relevant data; comparison of previous data with current data; prioritization of the issues to be negotiated; coming up with probable options; determining the other party's expectations; formulating a negotiation plan and creating a meeting schedule.

When reviewing notes, it is important to note the tactics previously used when an agreement was reached, the main issues that came up and who the stakeholders were at the time.

Data collection involves ascertaining what the cost of labor is, the number of hours worked on average, comparison of income against expenditure and the cost of employees' leave.

As a nurse executive, you need to do your best to ensure negotiations are factual and not emotional. To start the negotiations, each party must make an opening statement, explaining what their expectations are. In negotiations, the parties involved should not initially state the position that they consider most reasonable or best for the other party. Instead, they should leave room to maneuver during the negotiations.

Handling of Grievances

Grievances include disputes regarding employment terms, sometimes where terms of the CBA have been violated or are being poorly implemented, or where one party feels the rules are being misinterpreted.

Any employees with a grievance are expected to present it to their immediate supervisors in written form. If the issue is beyond the authority of an immediate supervisor, the supervisor forwards it up the administrative ladder. In short, in trying to resolve a dispute, it is imperative that the institution's command chain is followed.

If a dispute reaches the top of the administrative ladder and is still not resolved, the next step is normally to forward the issue for arbitration by an impartial third party. Such an arbitrator expects to be presented with facts, and the decision he/she arrives at on the basis of those facts binds both of the parties involved in the dispute. Whenever a grievance is presented for arbitration, both parties should expect to share half of the cost of arbitration.

The National Labor Relations Board

The National Labor Relations Board (NLRB) is an agency of the federal government whose role is to safeguard the right of workers to form and join labor unions. It is important to note that even where employees are not members of any union, they are still protected by the NLRB. This means that the board's mandate extends even to nonprofit organizations.

NLRB Offices

This board has thirty-two offices regionally, with their roles well defined. One office, for example, provides a framework within which employees can organize and conduct their elections. Another investigates whenever there are allegations of unfair labor practices.

Whenever there is a dispute between employers and employees, the NLRB facilitates a settlement. The board has forty judges who work hand in hand with the NLRB to adjudicate labor-related cases.

It is important to note that not only are employers banned from dissuading employees from joining labor unions, but they are also required to display a notice detailing the rights of employees.

Principles and Styles of Communication

Among the issues nurse executives are required to be conversant with are principles of communication, which encompass active listening, reflective communication, two-way communication, the loop of feedback between sender and receiver, hiring interview and motivational interviewing.

Active Listening

When a person is actively listening to another, he/she not only pays attention but also carefully observes everything involving the communication including the person's body posture, demeanor and other forms of nonverbal communication.

An actively listening person also provides feedback, as opposed to letting the other person engage in a monologue. Giving feedback not only confirms that someone is paying interest, but it is also respectful. It is important to note that feedback does not have to be an opinion; it can also be a question or a gesture like a nod.

Empathy is the other major component of active listening. It involves indicating that you understand the person's feelings. If, for example, you tell a coworker, "I can imagine how disappointed you must be after being overlooked for the promotion," the statement communicates to the other person that you are sincerely empathetic to his/her situation.

Reflective Communication

Reflective communication is especially helpful when it leads the other person to appreciate the feelings he/she is experiencing, and which the person may not have considered. For example, if a person is complaining about the human resources manager not approving an unpaid leave of absence, yet two years ago human resources approved a similar leave for a colleague, you could say, "That appears like a double standard and is really upsetting you."

Such a remark shows the person how his/her feelings are coming across, and if those are not the actual feelings he/she has, then the person can rethink how to frame the complaint when venting. Reflective communication assists individuals to develop better attitudes towards others and to the things happening within their environment.

Two-Way Communication

In two-way communication, talk between two individuals is balanced so that both are equally voicing their opinions, volunteering information and asking questions without either person dominating the conversation.

Although the sender-receiver feedback loop is independently a mode of communication, it is also applicable in a balanced conversation like the two-way. Feedback is paramount in both cases.

Two-way communication in a hospital setup is evident in a conversation between nurses who are coworkers in a unit. This is described as horizontal communication. It can also be between a nurse executive and a nurse from the ICU, the pediatric ward or any of the other hospital units. The nurse executive is an administrator and senior to all those other nurses. When two-way communication is between a senior and someone junior, it is described as vertical or downward.

The Sender-Receiver Feedback Loop

The basis of this process of communication is the 1948 theory of information originated by Claude Shannon. Shannon singled out three steps as being necessary for effective communication: encoding, transmitting and decoding.

Encoding involves the person originating the message—the encoder—"encoding" it, meaning to compile the message in the desired form, such as writing it down on paper.

Transmitting involves sending the message with the aim of it reaching the intended recipient. There should be a channel through which to do this like email, phone, television, etc.

Decoding of the message is done by the message recipient, who attaches meaning to the message. The only way that the encoder knows if the message transmitted was given the intended meaning is when the decoder provides feedback. For this reason, feedback is very important in communication.

Two factors that can influence the decoding of a message are context and interference. The physical or psychological environment within which the message finds the decoder can have some influence on how he/she ascribes meaning. For example, a message received on a dance floor may be poorly received because of the noise.

Interference includes other factors, including external ones, with the capacity to impact or distort how the message is received or decoded. For example, a message received by a person who has just gotten news that he/she has failed an exam may be poorly decoded because of the negative emotions the person is experiencing at the time the message arrives.

Interviews for Staff Hiring

Effective communication is necessary when conducting interviews with the aim of hiring personnel. To ask appropriate questions, the individuals involved need to familiarize themselves with the job description, as well as the applicants' history.

It is also important that questions be prepared in advance and that all members of the panel have a copy of the questions.

The questions posed to job applicants should be related to the job advertised, and they should also conform to the laws of the state and federal law. This means that questions pertaining to the age of the interviewee, his/her ethnicity and anything else discriminatory is not permissible.

Motivational Interviewing

Motivational interviewing, as explained in the 1983 publication of the same title by Miller, is an approach that seeks to identify how ready the interviewee is to embrace change. It also helps the interviewer to devise strategies suitable for making the individual most effective in his/her role.

The questions the interviewer asks should not provide for one-word answers, but instead allow the candidate to express himself/herself in a broad manner. Affirmation should be given where a candidate's strengths are noted. Reflective listening works well when conducting motivational interviewing.

Styles of Communication

Nurse executives need to understand different styles of communication, and must be able to employ each of them as the situation calls for it. The major communication styles include persuasive, assertive, passive, aggressive and passive-aggressive.

Persuasive Communication

Persuasive communication involves trying to convince someone to accept something, do something or trust something. This communication style is very important in the field of health care, as nurses and other service providers are continually faced with patients who have fears regarding their health and the best way to address it.

The most significant steps in persuasive communication include understanding a listener, capturing the listener's attention, cultivating credibility with the listener, pinpointing accruing benefits and using suitable body language.

Assertive Communication

Assertive communication involves the expression of an opinion in a firm and direct manner, with a speaker's actions matching his/her words. Many of the statements in assertive communication begin with "I," like "I'd like to review this or that" or "I'd like to start with this and end with that," and so on.

It is important to note that assertiveness in communication is normally accompanied by a show of respect. In fact, often, when people engage in assertive communication, they involve the other party by using cooperative statements like "What is your opinion on this?"

Passive Communication

In passive communication, the individual communicates in a manner that is not direct, either in words or in body language. Often people communicating passively do not contribute anything of significance in a conversation, and they are often unwilling to indicate their stance on the issue under discussion.

One of the reasons people communicate in a passive way is the belief that their opinions do not matter. Sometimes such people manifest nervousness in the course of conversation, avoiding making eye contact or fidgeting. Because such people like to avoid conflict, they sometimes laugh even when they disagree with what has been said. In the short-term, the person engaged in passive communication manages to avoid conflict.

Aggressive Communication

While some major qualities of assertiveness are also found in aggressive communication, the latter lacks the important element of respect for the listener, which is central in assertive communication.

An aggressive communicator gets the other party to agree with him/her by bullying; this style often leads to the communicator being resented and causes anxiety. Other qualities of aggressive communication include sarcasm, insults, mid-sentence interruptions and intrusion into the other person's space.

Often the body language of a person engaged in aggressive communication is upright and with feet apart, hands on hips; aggressive communicators are often seen pointing a finger or forming a fist. The only advantage to such aggressiveness is getting what you want. The other person does not benefit from the communication.

Passive-Aggressive Communication

When communication is passive-aggressive, not only is direct communication lacking, but there are negative emotions beneath what is in clear view. The person communicating is not only angry but also resentful. It is a big disadvantage to deal with a communicator who is passive-aggressive because while the person may appear to agree with your point of view, once the conversation is finished, the person may undermine you and obstruct your efforts.

Passive-aggressive people have the tendency to air their discontent with other people, but hardly say a word regarding their genuine feelings to the individual concerned. They seek support from other people in indirect ways, and sometimes they are inclined to sabotage the efforts of others. Passive-aggressive people rarely own up to the negative feelings they harbor towards others.

Cultural Elements of Communication

It is important that nurse executives understand how to factor in cultural values of individual communities, and their modes of behavior in communication. For example, among the Hmong of Southeast Asia, decisions affecting members of the family are made by the eldest male family member. For that reason, and taking into account the respect given to that individual, the nurse should avoid giving information pertaining to the patient to any other person. Instead, the nurse should inquire who the right person is to discuss matters concerning the patient with, and when communicating with that family representative, the nurse should avoid looking him in the eye.

When dealing with patients of Mexican descent, nurses should be very clear about time, because the culture tends not to take time very seriously. For instance, a nurse should avoid asking a Mexican patient to see him/her in the office "after lunch," because the patient may consider that to be past 3 p.m. Instead, the nurse should specify the time, like 1:45.

Chapter 3: Human Resource Management – Skills

Models of Staffing in Nursing (Staffing Fundamentals)

The nursing models used in the US include

- primary care nursing
- team nursing
- modular nursing
- total patient care
- functional nursing
- patient-centered care
- twelve-bed hospital
- nurse-patient ratio-based
- acuity-based
- and RN skill mix.

It is important to note that when the term RN skill mix is used as a staffing model, it is in reference to the ratio of registered nurses providing direct patient care in an institution as opposed to handling just supervisory duties.

How to Calculate RN Skill Mix

Suppose a unit in Hospital XYZ has budgeted for an FTE staff of 50. Thirty-five of them are RNs, 8 of them LVNs, while 7 are UAPs. What is the RN skill mix?

Answer

Number of RNs = 35

Total number of nurses = 35 + 8 + 7 = 50

The RN skill mix = 35:50 = 7:10

The RN skill mix in this case can be expressed as 70 percent.

One important factor that makes analysis of the skill mix important is that if it is extremely low, the service provided to patients may be below par, and if it is extremely high, staffing costs might end up being excessive.

Workflow

Nurse executives are required to be conversant with workflow, including how to design it on the basis of care delivered and the size of the population being served.

In this regard, nurse executives should familiarize themselves with

- workflow mapping
- interdisciplinary teams
- case management and associated models
- disease management
- throughput
- assignment of staff and scheduling
- and scheduling models.

Development of Policies & Procedures

The role of nurse executives in health institutions demands that they be well versed in ways to develop policies and procedures, which help to ensure an institution is compliant with applicable regulations and standards the profession has set. Along the same lines, the nurse executive is responsible for ensuring that the integrity of the organization is maintained.

To fulfill this role adequately, nurse executives are expected to learn about the legal requirements, those of a regulatory nature, all the applicable policies and procedures, as well as work-related standards. It is crucial that nurse executives stay updated on the changes happening in the health profession, including any changes in regulations, and share that information with staff in a timely manner. This means nurse executives must attend workshops and seminars where health matters are being discussed, whether facilitated by federal or state agencies, or professional bodies.

Utilization of Resources

Since nurse executives are responsible for handling many issues pertaining to staff performance, it is important that they understand the best ways to utilize resources available to health-care institutions, including human resources.

Cross-Training

One way staff can be better utilized is by ensuring training provides them with diverse skills and that they are given room to test those skills in different sections of the health-care institution. This way, when one unit has a shortage, it can easily be supported by staff from a different unit.

This is referred to as cross-training. It is geared toward allowing staff members to be able to handle different jobs in the workplace. Such proficiency is enhanced when staff members are rotated from time to time.

Accordion Schedule

The accordion schedule is one that nurse executives use to ensure that all staff positions are filled on a daily basis, even if someone is absent from work.

Job Description

A job description details what a particular position entails in terms of responsibilities and the skills a person should possess in order to be considered a good fit for the position.

A job description includes the title of the job, employment location and a short description of that position. If the position warrants it, the description can include the office holder the successful candidate is expected to report to.

It is important that the job responsibilities be detailed in the job description in order of their priority. A condensed summary of ten to fifteen points is appropriate.

The job description should address required academic qualifications and working experience. Major benefits that come with the position should be mentioned, including length of vacation and retirement benefits.

Other important features of a job description include the salary or its range, and any applicable CBA. It is important that job descriptions be written using language that is not biased against any gender. If the job advertisement is placed online, it is crucial that effective key words be used, so that the ad can reach as many people as possible.

Human Resource Principles

Among the principles associated with human resources are assistance and counseling given to employees, determination of compensation rates and benefits, coaching and others.

Assistance & Counseling for Employees

Many organizations provide employee benefits packages. These are generally termed Employee Assistance Programs (EAPs). Although varied, some benefits apply across the board, like counseling services. For example, any employees with PTSD are provided with special help. Other issues that lead to individuals being offered special help include abuse of illicit substances; domestic abuse; work-related stress and that of an emotional nature; financial and legal problems and life-based events like childbirth, loss of kin, ailment or disability.

Seeking assistance from an EAP is voluntary, and it is free of charge if no referral is required. For the purposes of encouraging employees to seek assistance when in need, the information revealed is kept confidential. In some cases, providers may recommend that help be extended to an employee's family. In addition to the EAPs set up by the federal government, others can be found at the state level and in the private business sector.

Determination of Compensation

When a job position is created, there must be a way to determine its cost, which is the commensurate salary and the costs linked to all other benefits. The salary should reflect the market trends with regards to the industry and the geographical region.

The most preferred ways of quoting a salary for a given position include dollars, as a range, as negotiable or added incentives. Once the salary is indicated in precise dollars, no room for negotiation is left, even if the applicant has some additional skills besides those stated in the job description.

When the salary is indicated as a range, there is room for potential bias, and so there needs to be a rubric to help determine the best number for every applicant. This should take into account an applicant's experience in terms of years, special skills or continuing education credits.

Incentives are ordinarily given when a position has a shortage of qualified applicants; in short, when qualified individuals are hesitant to apply. Such incentives can be provided in the form of a bonus at the time of hiring.

When it comes to negotiable salaries, this may involve individuals carrying out similar tasks but being paid widely varying salaries. This can lead to a company being seen as having a recruitment bias.

Work-Related Benefits

Benefits are important to potential and existing employees and therefore should be taken seriously by the administration. Important benefits include leave times, insurance coverage, childcare, retirement benefits, forgiveness of student loans, provision of transport, etc.

Employee Performance Management

Competency validation and performance appraisals are an important part of performance management. Competency validation can be achieved through surveys, evidence of daily work, checklists, observation, testing or presentations. Performance appraisals are assessments of the employee that determine overall contribution to the company's values and objectives.

Performance management entails the assessment of employees' performance for the sake of ensuring the success of an organization's goals. Although individual employees are assessed, the performance of specified groups and the institution in general is also evaluated. There are three major steps necessary for successful performance management.

1. **Development of a Plan of Performance**

The administration must carry out a review of a given job description in collaboration with the target employee(s) and then agree on the outcomes expected by the end of a given period. These should be compiled into three to five goals. Besides setting goals and timelines, the parties should also agree on how success in meeting these goals should be measured.

2. **Employee Coaching**

The intention of coaching is to assist employees in their efforts to meet established goals. Such assistance can be in the form of positive or negative feedback. There may be a need to schedule regular meetings to facilitate such feedback.

When coaching an employee, it is best to focus on matters of priority, suitable behavior and constructive criticism.

3. **Performance Assessment (Appraisal)**

Assessing individuals' or groups' performances needs to be done on an annual basis at the minimum. Such assessments should be a joint exercise between employee(s) and employer(s).

Employee Engagement Strategies

Culture, transparency, recognition, accountability, enforcement, feedback and professioanl development are all part of employee engagement. These areas are covered in detail in the following sections.

The Culture of the Organization

An institution's administration expects employees to do what is expected of them at all times, including meeting their set targets on schedule. When these expectations are not met, often the employees are taken to task. Nevertheless, it has been found that there are better ways of enhancing performance than blaming the employees, and one of them involves adopting what is termed a "just culture."

Just Culture

An employer who adopts a just culture is not quick to blame an employee who makes an error or fails to meet certain expectations. Instead, the employer sees the bigger picture, trying to determine organizational shortcomings that may have led to the employee's error. In short, in a just culture, the employer appreciates that, often, errors happen because of faults in the system. Those errors must be corrected in order for employees to be able to do their work properly.

In a hospital environment, for example, some system deficiencies that may be an underlying cause for employees' inefficiencies include too much overtime, unclear orders, understaffing, poor labeling of equipment, etc.

In short, the main feature of a just culture is the focus on streamlining a system as opposed to trying the change the behavior of an individual. To that end, the culture seeks to differentiate between three major features: human error, risky behavior and reckless behavior.

Human Error

Employers should show some consideration and try to establish the reason employees may have made mistakes. Management should address existing processes and procedures, and if necessary, arrange for in-service training or any other relevant on-the-job training for employees. Also, if considered helpful, procedures could be modified to make them easier to remember and execute.

Risky Behavior

Employees who have a tendency to take unwarranted risks should be coached appropriately. They should also be given incentives to reduce their appetite for risky actions. Also, considering that some employees may not be easily incentivized, measures should be put in place to serve as disincentives. Disincentives may be punitive in nature.

Reckless Behavior

Behavior is considered careless or reckless when a person knows what should be done yet chooses to do something different, irrespective of the outcome. To correct such behavior, action of a remedial nature may be taken, or punitive measures may also be enacted.

The Need for Transparency

Matters that are crucial to transparency in the workplace include disclosure of information, clarity in disseminating information and communication of information with accuracy.

In this regard, it is imperative that every individual working in an organization be informed on the things that do and do not work. Employees must be encouraged to give their input on the basis of the information they have. It is also advisable for the administration to be receptive to questions and to show appreciation for employees who volunteer to air their concerns by rewarding these individuals for their honesty.

Issues of transparency may include employees' salaries, ownership of the organization and specific transactions made by the organization. Such issues are easily communicated when an organization makes use of councils through which employees communicate any ideas they have. Organizations like these consider it important to share governance with their staff, considering their employees to be their partners, and all cadres have representatives in these councils.

For transparency to be successful, it is crucial for senior administrative personnel to act in a supportive manner. They should, for example, be prepared to provide answers to questions posed by the employees. They also should not be secretive about the organization's yield or investment returns. When there is a matter that is likely to affect employees, senior administrative personnel should be open about it, irrespective of whether the employees are likely to be impacted positively or adversely.

It is also important that every organization have a communication board that shares key information in a manner easily accessible to employees. Also, organizations should get into the habit of holding meetings with employees on a regular basis, allowing individuals time to share ideas and hear updates.

The Command Chain

There is a set standard of leadership adhered to by health-care institutions; one that ensures there is both a clearly defined command chain and accountability.

The hierarchy of the command chain has the institution's governing body at the helm, and immediately below is the chief executive officer (CEO). Immediately below the CEO comes the nurse executive, who is followed along the command chain by senior managers. Department heads then follow, and immediately below them are staff leaders, some of whom are elected by employees and others who are appointed. Nurse leaders can be found around this level, and then there are other staff members who provide support services.

It is important to note that the governing body is answerable for the care provided to the patients, even though the direct providers of the services are professional members of staff who include physicians and nurses, laboratory technicians and other staff. The governing body has the mandate to determine the authority structure and to spell out the scope and extent of responsibility for every employee within the health institution.

The Organizational Chart

Every health institution should have an organizational chart that pictorially depicts the command chain. It also should demonstrate the relationships that exist among different units of the organization and departments. The most popular organizational charts are hierarchical. This means command is via a top-down structure.

Matrix Format

The three charts are defined in terms of formats: matrix format, horizontal format and committee structure. Matrix has management at the very top, and the departments that follow below are all equal in authority. If the organization has units but not departments, those also have a similar level of authority in a matrix format.

Horizontal Format

Horizontal format, though similar to the matrix, has a less definitive top authority; the units or departments that come below are almost autonomous.

Committee Structure

Although authority is hierarchical here too, power is placed in the hands of committees rather than individuals. As such, there is an executive committee at the helm, followed immediately below by subcommittees, responsible for overseeing different departments and projects. The exact layout of this structure may have small variations among the institutions that use it.

Ad Hoc Committees

Ad hoc committees are formed to accomplish a particular purpose, and once that purpose has been fulfilled, the ad hoc committee is no longer needed. Whereas the other committees that oversee departments are permanent, ad hoc ones are temporary.

The Control Span

The number of people that report to a member of staff within an organization is said to constitute that member's span of control. It is important to define this span where the organization has a hierarchical command chain.

The control span, or the number of people to be supervised, is normally wide where the work being performed is mainly of a routine nature; thus there is not much to direct. The situation is different when the tasks being performed are complex, often being varied in nature; hence the control span is narrow.

How to Determine the Best Control Span

The best way to determine the best size of a control span is to take the organization's size into account as well as the nature of skills the employees have, the culture the organization has built over time, the nature of training supervisors have received and the responsibilities various supervisors have.

Policies & Procedures and their Enforcement

Policies and procedures help an organization to run smoothly because it is through them that all employees know what is expected of them.

How to Develop Policy

An institution's mission statement must always be considered when trying to develop or modify policies and procedures. Policies are guidelines designed to formally assist in the making of decisions and ensure there is consistency in the manner actions are taken. Policies should be broad, general and easily understood. It is important that the wording used in a policy be simple and clear enough for any member of staff to understand.

The formulators of a policy should seek input from every sector of the organization. The policy must then receive approval from the board in order for it to be applicable. While some institutions compile a manual explaining their policies, others only provide them online.

How to Develop Procedures

Unlike policies, procedures are detailed. They spell out every step of a process in sequential order, and for that reason, it is important that procedures only be established after adequate research has been done, and the suggested practices are confirmed as being appropriate for the organization.

The process of developing a procedure begins with stating its purpose. Individuals best suited to develop that procedure are then identified. Another important component of procedure development is the compilation of a list of materials and equipment deemed necessary for executing the procedure, and a list of the steps that need to be followed. Procedures are sometimes specific to individual units; for example, there may be a procedure specific to the administration of chemotherapy.

How to Monitor Compliance

Compliance monitoring can only be meaningful if staff has been educated on existing policies and procedures. After ensuring that employees have a good understanding of these, the administration should state clearly that it is imperative that the policies and procedures be followed to the letter. It is also important to encourage staff members to identify any procedures or policies which need to be revised.

Monitoring compliance can be formal as well as informal, the latter being done through interviews and general discussions. Staff members must be made aware of the repercussions of not adhering to the institution's policies and procedures.

When a staff member fails to comply with any policy or procedure, the person should be retrained. If repeat noncompliance is noted, more serious action should be taken, especially if the person's noncompliance puts patients or the institution at risk.

Feedback on Policy & Procedure Success

It should be an annual practice to review the policies and procedures in place, always with a view to matching them with the prevailing needs of the organization. An interdisciplinary team should participate in such reviews, and it is advisable to seek feedback from members of staff. The staff should be made aware that there is room for policy change, and that their input would be appreciated. This can be done through emails or meetings, or any other form of communication deemed appropriate by the organization.

When it comes to modification of procedures, the questions should be asked: Is there evidence that procedures are working optimally? Do these procedures follow best global practices?

Modifying & Expanding Job Descriptions

It is important for roles to be assessed and modified as changes occur in the health-care sector. Some roles will be altered or expanded from what they used to be, sometimes due to the necessity to add new skills to a position. A good example is the requirement that nurses be computer literate so that they are able to use electronic health records (EHRs).

An established job's description may need to be changed when tasks are added to it. Before making the final determination to change a job description, it is important to make comparisons with other positions within and beyond the organization. It is also advisable to have discussions pertaining to such potential changes, not only with supervisors at the unit level but also with ordinary staff and other stakeholders.

One of the advantages of having a suitable job description is the potential of attracting suitable candidates for the position. At the same time, when the person's job description is suitable, it is relatively easy to determine the nature of training and/or evaluating an individual member of staff requires.

Professional Development

Professional development includes training of a specialized nature or one that is task-oriented, continuing nurse education, academic advancement and certification. During specialized training, the person is taught how to carry out defined tasks like monitoring cardiac activity. Often such training is done in-house, where the staff member in training observes an expert at work over a period of time. This is termed job shadowing. Other times individual staff members are taught by their peers.

Team Performance Management

Team performance management consists of essentially four elements: negotiation, communication, collaboration and conflict management. These areas are dicussed below.

How to Approach Negotiation

Nurses are expected to be familiar with various approaches of effective negotiation, which may be either formal or informal. Salary negotiations, for example, are formal in nature. When nurses are discussing as a team how they should go about doing things, like adjusting their departmental work schedule, the negotiations generally take place informally.

Ordinarily, the nature of negotiations depends on what they are meant to achieve, their purpose and who the participants are. There is a range of approaches to choose from as far as negotiations are concerned, and they include competition, accommodation, avoidance, compromise and collaboration.

Concepts of Negotiation

There are two major negotiation concepts, distributive and integrative. Negotiation is distributive when it is a win-lose situation, and it is integrative when it is a win-win situation. In these situations, there is room for bargaining.

Strikes as a Form of Communication

Strikes are normally held after negotiations have hit a stalemate; the wronged party, like the employees, goes on strike as a means of trying to influence the employer to give in to demands.

The major types of strikes are unfair labor practices, unprotected strikes, economic strikes and sympathy strikes.

Processes of Communication Supportive of Patient Safety

The major processes that support patient safety include documentation, situation-background-assessment-recommendation, bedside reporting, incident reporting and reporting of sentinel events.

Forms & Importance of Written Communication

Nurse executives need to be aware of situations where communication should be put in writing. Among those instances is presenting a formal or official proposal, sending out an advertisement, creating brochures and writing official letters. Also, after all negotiations and other processes have been completed, the final contract must be in written form.

It is worth noting that with changing technology, emails and documents sent electronically are increasingly being accepted as replacements for written communication. Whatever the manner of communication chosen, a nurse executive needs to be conscious of the purpose and structure the communication appropriately.

Scripting

Scripting involves preparing a message ahead of time. This ensures that all the people involved in communicating the message have the same information. An example of an instance when scripting comes in handy is during patient orientation by members of staff.

Scripting begins with deciding a purpose, followed by wording the actual message to be delivered. This means the opening should contain the crucial topic and script purpose, like this: “Mr. King, we would like to revise the preparatory steps for your colonoscopy.” Ultimately, the script should serve as a guide and not be recited word for word.

Verbal Communication Methods

Verbal communication has traditionally been face-to-face, as well as over landlines or cell phones. However, although emails and ordinary mail are considered tools of formal communication, they are sometimes used informally to add a personal touch.

The internet has also provided myriad tools for verbal communication, including video calls, videoconferencing, web pages, social media and other internet channels.

Nonverbal Communication Methods

Nonverbal communication encompasses eye contact, tone of voice, gestures, posture and touch.

How to Facilitate Collaboration for an Optimal Outcome

In order for the results of collaboration among individuals or teams to be the best possible, team building is important.

The Essence of Team Building

For proper team building, which is meant to enhance collaboration and lead to improved performance, individuals must be given a chance to define what their role is. This stage is considered the initial interaction.

Issues pertaining to power are also dealt with when team members determine who the team leader should be. The next stage is organizing, where the methods to be followed in performing a task are agreed upon.

Soon members of the team develop rapport as they interact in the process of working, and that stage is referred to as team identification. During this stage, every member wants the other to succeed.

The final phase is excellence, where the team's success is evident. Excellence is reached as a result of:

- suitable leadership
- commitment from team members
- clarity of goals set
- high level of set standards
- recognition from external parties
- sense of collaboration
- and team members being collectively committed to the whole process.

Types of Groups

For the purposes of communication, various types of groups are formed.

Groups of Form

Groups of form are homogenous, with members specifically selected to be part of them; for example, the staff of the emergency department.

Other groups are heterogeneous, with members who are diverse in age, gender and roles. Another type, the mixed group, comprises members with something in common, while at the same time differing in aspects like gender or age.

The major characteristic of a "closed" group is that it is not open to new members. A group is said to be open when members and group leadership can change.

Groups of Purpose

Groups can also be formed according to their purpose, such as to accomplish a given task or to teach new staff how tasks in a particular unit should be handled.

A group can be formed to provide therapy or personal support to members of staff struggling with their personal or professional lives.

Structure of Teams

The structure of a team is crucial in ensuring success. Structure involves selecting people with the right skill set, who complement one another. Other considerations when creating a team include the team size, performance goals, the approach and accountability, which should be collective.

Additional Matters Pertaining to Team Operations

Other areas a nurse executive should be familiar with include:

- forming teams to ensure the institution's performance is constantly improving
- forming teams to handle disciplinary issues
- overseeing phases of group processes
- responsibility for stages of group formation or development, like Tuckman's stages of group development
- and leveraging diversity.

Nurse executives should also learn how to select appropriate methods of communication and how to identify their audience.

Conflict Management

It is crucial for nurse executives to be able to handle conflict in a manner that does not affect health-care delivery adversely.

Approaches to Conflict

Nurse executives must be conversant with the major approaches to conflict resolution, which include one of the parties being either accommodating, skilled in avoiding conflict or helping the parties involved to collaborate.

Other approaches that nurse executives need to learn include

- compromise involving both parties,
- confronting issues
- one party forcing the way forward
- negotiating
- being reassuring

- active problem-solving
- or withdrawing of one party and ceasing to be part of the conflict.

Steps Crucial to Resolving Conflict

Besides learning the steps that are crucial to resolving conflicts, nurse executives should know the distinction between ethical conflicts and those of a clinical nature. They should also understand the difference between positive and negative aspects of conflict.

Conflict Types & Levels

It is also important that nurse executives understand how to distinguish between intrapersonal and interpersonal conflict.

Alongside conflict levels, it is important also to understand the major conflict types— those pertaining to personal relationships, tasks or processes.

Nurse executives should also be conversant with how to handle defensiveness. They should know if parties in conflict need to be separated, whether the conflict requires suppressing or ignoring and/or if the solution should be indirectly implemented.

Organizational Conflicts

Conflicts are deemed organizational when they erupt within the institution, like those that may occur within a particular hospital. Some of the reasons such conflicts occur revolve around power. Others are due to poor communication or varying goals within the institution.

Other reasons for organizational conflicts revolve around allocation of resources and roles in relation to the work allocated to someone. Some conflicts are interpersonal in nature. A nurse executive is expected to know the best approach to each type of conflict in order to restore order in the health-care institution.

Chapter 4: Quality and Safety – Knowledge

When considering models of professional practice, collaboration among different disciplines must be taken into account. Such collaboration helps to enhance the benefits for both the patients and their families.

Change Management

For any change to be meaningful, it needs to happen both on an individual and organizational level. The steps individuals need to take in order to be effective in executing change are represented by the acronym ADKAR, which stands for awareness, desire, knowledge, ability and reinforcement.

The person in charge of managing change must:

- be aware that a change is necessary
- fight the fear of having things change
- genuinely desire change
- be equipped with the relevant knowledge and skills to carry out the needed change
- be able to coach others who are expected to help drive the change
- be able to reinforce the new change
- and keep others from reverting to old ways of doing things.

Nurse executives need to be conversant with:

1. Kurt Lewin's theory of change that Edgar Schein later modified
2. Kurt Lewin's force-field analysis
3. The six distinct phases that planned change undergoes
4. The seven distinct phases that planned change undergoes as explained in the 1958 publication by Lippitt, Watson and Westley
5. Kotter's eight-step theory of change
6. The transtheoretical model of change
7. The McKenzie 7S Framework
8. The Nudge theory
9. Bridge's model of transition.

Culture of Safety

One of the areas covered under safety culture is risk management, which involves identifying risk, analyzing it, preventing future risks and assessing the corrective measures put in place.

Other areas include stratification of risks; accountability; employee involvement; technologies for safety of employees; technologies for safety of patients; Radio Frequency Identification; patient safety programs and environmental risks and hazards.

Risk Management

Risk management involves identifying, monitoring and controlling risks in the workplace. These risks can be medical in nature or related to employee dynamics. Qualitative assessments can be done through charts and quantitative assessments can be done via computer programs. Risks can be avoided, accepted, mitigated, or escalated to management.

How to Ensure a Work Environment is Healthy

The most crucial elements of effective leadership, as per the ANA, are safety, empowerment and satisfaction.

Environmental Safety

Safety encompasses the environment in its entirety. The institution must have fire escape routes, good air quality and sufficient lighting and heating. To enhance safety, employees should be well trained on isolation protocols and on how to use equipment like lifts effectively.

The environment should also be free from bullying and all other forms of violence.

Staff Empowerment

Good leadership requires that members of staff be accorded a degree of autonomy that matches the respective positions they hold. It also requires that employees be given opportunities to further their learning and enhance their growth.

Staff Satisfaction

Employers in the health-care sector need to ensure that their employees are well remunerated and have reasonable working hours with flexible schedules. This leads to staff having positive attitudes, thereby rendering better-quality service.

Chapter 5: Quality and Safety – Skills

The two main sections in this chapter are Continuous Process Improvement and Research & Practice Methods. This chapter also covers systems theories.

Continuous Process Improvement

For the purpose of this guide, continuous process improvement includes the PDSA Cycle, Lean Six Sigma and Root Cause Analysis.

PDSA Cycle

The PDSA cycle is also called the Deming cycle and was deveoped in the early 1900s by Walter A. Shewhart and W. Edwards Deming. The cycle explains that we should plan, do, study and act upon our observations. This is repetitive cycle that nurses would apply to the employee management, risk management and data management.

Lean Six Sigma

Lean six sigma is a process improvement methodology that is normally used in manufacturing environments. The six stages are: recognize, define, measure, analyze, improve and control.

Root Cause Analysis

Root cause anlaysis attempts to fix issues by eliminating or mitigating the sources of issues, instead of trying to treat the symptoms of an issue. It is often paired up with preventive measures.

Research & Practice Based on Evidence

The second part of knowledge management involves evidence-based research and practice.

Research-Subject Protection

It is important that nurse executives be versed with the role of the Institutional Review Board (IRB) and the laws pertaining to the protection of people who serve as subjects of research, including the HHI, and the FDA's code.

Research & Practice Techniques

Nurse executives are expected to conduct reviews of relevant literature, beginning with searching different databases for helpful articles. They should also be able to do research to find appropriate literature, both current and historical; work with SQL, a computer language, and know the steps to be followed in critical reading, which is important if research is to be properly evaluated.

Other areas nurse executives are expected to be knowledgeable about include the format termed PICOT, which guides how quantitative questions are designed. PICOT stands for patient or population, intervention or indicator, comparison or control, and time.

Nurse executives also need to be skilled in developing methods of study as well as design. They must know how to carry out descriptive research as well as co-relational research. They should be able to conduct case-control studies, cohort studies, cross-sectional studies, quasi-experimental and experimental research and be able to link any evidence to preferable outcomes.

Other areas nurse executives are expected to be conversant with include sourcing and using quantitative and qualitative data, data management in general and the fundamental steps in any research process.

Improvement of Performance through Research

Nurse executives must be skilled in performance enhancement, and for this to be possible, they need to understand crucial elements of research like PI and its performance models, CQI and TQM, as well as evidence-based practice.

Culture Creation & Advocacy for Research Resources

Whereas different people may be involved in carrying out research in an institution, nurse executives are expected to advocate for them. They also should consciously work towards developing a suitable culture for the institution.

These goals can be achieved by forming a journal club, which normally comprises professionals. The club meets on a regular basis, and the focus is on reviewing scientific journals and other professional literature that can help improve staff performance as well as that of the institution as a whole.

Nurse executives must be knowledgeable about writing grants to secure resources for the purposes of upgrading systems and developing modern programs to help improve performance.

Nurse executives should also help in the formation of an interdisciplinary council whose main role is to promote and support research. Because such a council is formal in nature, it should have a charter.

Other areas nurse executives are expected to be knowledgeable about include how to evaluate newfound knowledge and research findings, incorporating these into the practices of the institution.

Knowledge Management Through Innovation

Candidates for the nurse executive exam need to study the various ways through which innovation is carried out in the field of clinical practice, including how to diffuse innovations, which revolves around the adoption of new concepts.

Other important areas include:

- how to adopt innovations
- factors on which the success of innovation depends
- leadership in the context of innovation
- how to develop a framework to help with the implementation of innovations
- how to institute a pilot program
- how to leverage an institution's diversity
- and how to evaluate and apply technology.

Systems Theories

Nurse executives are required to learn about the systems theory, under which falls the Total-Person Systems Model, the Complex Adaptive Theory, Bertalanffy Systems Theory, the Contingency Theory, the Scientific Management Theory & Motivation Theory.

Innovation Management Theory

Innovation management involves comparing organic systems to those that are mechanistic. The general idea is that one should think broadly about the choices available on how to run an institution because each of them has a unique culture, context and product.

According to Stalker & Burns' theory, every institution should have a management structure that suits it, with managers designing a system that corresponds to the environment within which the organization exists.

Systems are considered organic when their conditions are subject to change and mechanistic when their conditions are stable.

Learning Organizations

Learning organizations continually undergo transformations, and they facilitate learning and education for their staff. Although these institutions easily adapt to changes, their success is dependent on how willing their members are to learn and how empowered they then become.

There are five distinct disciplines of a learning institution: personal mastery, mental models, shared vision, team learning and systems thinking. Personal mastery involves a person creating favorable outcomes, while mental model is about how a person's mindset affects his/her decisions and actions.

Shared vision is about individuals sharing with others within their group their own visions regarding the future. In team learning, there is a sharing of knowledge and skills in a bid to improve the group's capacity. Meanwhile, systems thinking is about viewing the institution holistically, with its departments and units being interrelated.

Nurse executives are required to familiarize themselves with the X & Y theories of 1960. These are two theories created by the same person, Douglas McGregor, yet they conflict. While theory X views workers generally as unmotivated and averse to working, theory Y suggests that it is possible to motivate workers and to help them enjoy working.

CQI

Continuous Quality Improvement (CQI) emphasizes an institution's systems rather than the individuals in the institution. In CQI, there is an appreciation of both internal and external customers, the former being staff members and the latter being patients.

TQM

Total Quality Management (TQM) is a philosophy regarding quality management, which emphasizes the need to include all stakeholders within an institution when finding solutions to problems, without any inclination to assign blame.

FOCUS

FOCUS is an acronym for find, organize, clarify, uncover and start. This is a performance enhancement model that is applied when facilitating change. In *find*, attempts are made to identify any area of the institution that is not working optimally; in *organize*, individuals familiar with the problem are identified and brought together as a team.

In *clarify*, team members brainstorm what should be done to alleviate the problem. In the *uncover* phase, efforts are made to establish why the problem arose in the first place, or why the affected process has not succeeded. The *start* phase, which is the last, is where a decision is made as to the exact point where the necessary corrective measures should begin.

Other issues candidates need to study include the PDCA cycle, otherwise referred to as PDSA; the Accelerated Rapid-Cycle Change approach; Juran's QIP; Six Sigma; DMAIC; Lean; Lean Six Sigma; FADE; RCA; Is-Is Not method; the five Whys; FMEA and Tracer Methodology.

Measures of Processes & Outcomes

The areas to be studied under these measures include clinical outcome, which involves patient outcomes in relation to patient populations, prioritization in alignment with the mission of the institution and other factors; the finance department as a resource center for valuable data; safety standards and areas requiring safety-related interventions; assessment of patients' satisfaction and assessment of employees' satisfaction.

Creation of a Continuous Performance Enhancement Culture

Proper commitment is required from nurse executives if a culture of continually improving performance is to become a foundational part of an institution. Nurse executives need to be ready to involve staff at every level in pinpointing the areas where improvements are crucial and getting everyone to make performance improvement their major focus.

Trending Internally & Benchmarking Externally

Trending internally involves comparing between one region or a particular population's internal rates, with another region or population. A good example is the comparison of the infection rate in an institution's ICU with those of other institutions.

Benchmarking externally involves analyzing data from beyond the institution and then comparing the result to what happens within the institution. A good example is analyzing and monitoring of infections that patients develop while hospitalized at the national level and then comparing that with the internal rate of such infections.

Data Dissemination within the Organization

It is important that data is disseminated at every level of the institution if performance is to be enhanced and for everyone to work towards the same institutional goals.

Areas that nurse executives need to understand under data dissemination include analyses of reports on performance productivity; data dissemination methods; media through which to disseminate research findings and other observations; digital dashboards and the balanced scorecard, as designed by Kaplan & Norton.

Chapter 6: Business Management – Knowledge and Skills

Nurse executives should be able to manage matters of finance and budgeting for a health institution and must have an understanding of how institutions obtain revenue and spend it.

Management of Finances

Nurse executives need to be able to monitor how money is being spent, analyze expenditures and submit reports.

Normally, finance-based planning, which is part of an institution's strategic plan, covers a period of a year. The intent of financial planning is to ensure any expenditures always lead to the best results, whether in the form of revenues or anticipated output.

Objectives of Financial Planning

The objectives of financial planning include the development of plans comprising records of quantities, enabling financial activities to be evaluated, control of costs incurred and making available information that increases awareness about costs.

It is important that an institution's budget reflects the expected daily financial activity. This should also be integrated with the vision the institution has, alongside the organization's mission, objectives and overall goals. Also, everyone with some interest in the budget should be allowed to participate in the planning. Monitoring of financial performance should be an ongoing activity, so as to enable feedback and subsequently provide an opportunity for modifications to be made as needed.

Management of Budgets

Managing a budget should be done on a continuous basis, as it is the best way of ensuring the targets set in terms of financial expenditures are met, ensuring that such expenditures and their corresponding outputs correspond to the strategic goals of the institution.

Budget management entails accountability, control of expenditures, monitoring to ensure costs align to the benchmarks of best practices, development of corrective measures where variances are noted, utilization of a scorecard that involves both quantitative and qualitative measures meant to manage costs, and recognition of quality, where rewards are set for reaching or exceeding benchmarks. Development of budgets is discussed at length later in this chapter.

Revenue Cycles

For a revenue cycle to be complete, it must start with the admission of a patient and end with the receiving of revenue. Managing the revenue-based cycle involves dealing with the capturing process, which means getting the billing done. Another aspect of revenue cycle management pertains to reimbursements for all services provided.

The major components of a revenue cycle are

1. Registration or preregistration
2. Billable services
3. Coding
4. Chargemaster
5. Capture
6. Submission
7. Resubmission or appeals
8. Collection.

The first step of registration is where information pertaining to Medicare, any other insurance firm or an individual responsible for the anticipated costs is noted. The patient is given an identifier at this stage. Next, billable services are rendered to the patient. In coding, each service rendered is assigned a diagnostic and billing code. It is important to ensure that the hospital's chargemaster is regularly updated, so that accurate information can be drawn at any time.

The capture stage is where any cost charged to the patient is documented and compiled into a bill. Step six is submission, when the payment claims are forwarded to the party responsible, either individuals or insurance companies. Resubmissions or appeals involve rectifying any rejected claims and then submitting them again for processing and payment. Remittance is the stage when payments are received and processed. The final stage of the revenue cycle is where any bills that are yet to be settled are referred to a collections agency.

Supply Expenditures

Supply expenditures refers to the money spent on acquisition of inventory, where inventory represents the equipment that an institution requires to function. Institutions are expected to perform inventory at least once every year. However, often, institutions have an automatic system where the process of ordering begins when the inventory on hand reaches a predetermined level.

There are, nevertheless, institutions that order inventory when items are almost depleted, and this is referred to as "just-in-time" ordering.

Institutions that follow this system of reordering consider it advantageous because they save money by not purchasing an excessive quantity of inventory. Still, it's best when a computerized inventory management system is used. Since usually the orders made are in small quantities, there is no bidding involved, and so a shorter time is spent to accomplish the process.

When working in a big institution, official bid forms are completed by the nurse responsible for the task of reordering, and detailed information is recorded. For example, the exact brand of medication required is indicated, along with the time supplies should have arrived. These requirements are sent to at least three different suppliers to give them a chance to submit their bids.

It is important to note that while many people expect the lowest bid to win, some institutions prefer to purchase inventory from suppliers with brand products as opposed to generic ones. Still, there are those that have standing arrangements with suppliers, and in such cases, there is no reason for inviting bidders. Others have such arrangements for lease of equipment, and in the short-term, these arrangements are reasonably inexpensive.

Expenditure on Labor

This addresses overtime expenses, which often significantly increases the employer's wage bill, owing to stipulations by the FLSA. Considering this law requires payment of wages at one and a half times the normal wage rate, sometimes that expenditure is equivalent to the amount the institution would have spent hiring an additional employee or hiring someone on a part-time basis. If labor expenditures keep exceeding the amount budgeted, the manager concerned risks receiving a poor rating during his/her annual performance appraisal.

There are dangers in having too much overtime, and these include a greater chance of the employees making errors or sustaining injuries because they are exhausted, and their level of concentration is adversely affected.

One way overtime can be avoided is by ensuring the workforce is large enough to handle the responsibilities of the organization. This includes having staff on call to cover any unanticipated absenteeism.

Allocation of Costs

It only becomes possible to allocate costs appropriately once a thorough cost analysis is done; such allocation is important if a budget is to be realistic. When costs are analyzed, it becomes clear what costs are consumed by what unit, with direct costs being categorized separately from indirect costs. Costs that are specific to the unit, like the salaries of nurses working in a particular unit, are direct costs.

For example, taking the ICU to be a cost center, if there are ten nurses expected to work in the ICU, then the salaries of six nurses are part of the ICU's direct costs. The cost of oxygen used for patients in that unit is also a direct cost. Costs incurred by the entire hospital, like electricity, are apportioned appropriately, with the unit that is the greatest user incurring the biggest share of that cost. Any costs of operation that warrant being shared among units are termed overheads.

ROI & Depreciation

ROI stands for return on investment. It involves the profit an institution makes compared to the amount of money invested, given as a percentage. To obtain ROI, you divide profit by cost and multiply the result by a hundred. Suppose Hospital ABC invested $500,000 and received a profit of $600,000. The ROI would be ($600,000 ÷ $500,000) x 100 = 1.2%.

Hospitals are normally expected to target a profit margin of 2 percent on average, which is narrow compared to conventional business organizations. The ROI is calculated in advance, and then returns from capital equipment are spread across the period of time such equipment is expected to last; depreciation of the equipment is spread over a similar period.

Depreciation means the amount of money by which the value of a given piece of equipment or other fixed asset is reduced every financial period. Calculating depreciation helps the institution in planning when next to buy new machinery or equipment, or when to develop new buildings or renovate existing ones.

Productivity in Health-Care Institutions

Productivity, a term commonly used in manufacturing, is the measure of an institution's performance, which is quantified by calculating how many units of output are produced for every unit of input spent.

Practically, productivity can be calculated by comparing money invested to number of hours worked. The comparison can also be between nurse hours and patient hospital days. Another way of calculating productivity is comparing staff nurses to the entire health institution's census.

Terms Used in Assessment of Productivity

There are other terms used in the manufacturing sector that have also found their way into the health industry, like those used in evaluating the institution's performance.

Marginal Productivity

Marginal productivity entails what the institution produces in units for every additional unit spent. This is important because it is imperative that an organization know when to stop spending on particular things, including staff. Normally, when there are additions to expenditure, like employing an extra nurse, output increases, such as the number of patients per day.

Nevertheless, there is a point beyond which the number of patients treated in one day cannot go, even if an additional nurse was hired. If this fact is ignored and an institution continues to employ nurses beyond that point, this will result in a profit loss. That point is known as diminishing returns.

Economies of Scale

Economies of scale is a term used in reference to a situation where items are purchased in bulk for the purpose of lowering the cost incurred per unit of that product. For example, a hospital will spend less on medicines when it orders large quantities that can be conveniently sourced from manufacturers or their major distributors. This is as opposed to buying medications in small quantities and consistently reordering. In the latter scenario, the hospital is likely to source the medicines from retail pharmacies at comparatively higher prices, and if it buys from wholesalers, they still cannot qualify for any meaningful discounts.

Short-Run & Long-Run

The terms short-run and long-run are used to indicate the length of time it takes for specified activities to be performed or certain achievements to be made. The short-run is the period during which inputs are expected to stay constant.

On the other hand, during the long-run it becomes necessary to make adjustments to all the inputs required.

Substitution

Substitution is used in reference to the replacement made of a different, more inexpensive input.

All the above terms are commonly used when evaluating how economically viable an institution is. This is because analyses of costs are done so as to assess how cost-effective particular processes and pieces of equipment are, the level of productivity from individual units and other such economic evaluations.

The running of an organization should be geared towards increasing revenue and reducing costs. If a hospital has no intention of charging more for its services, then it needs to cut down on its costs.

The Cost-Benefit Analysis

In cost-benefit analysis, the cost of performing a given event, on average, is compared to the gains attained; on the basis of that, it can be determined if such events are worthwhile in the future. If not, alternative events to fulfill the same need can be considered if the benefits are greater.

In the health sector, consider an instance where the CDC takes the cost of an infection on a surgical area to be $27,000, a figure arrived at after the cost for a surgical patient's twelve extra hospitalization days is calculated. If the hospital gets ten such surgical cases in one year, it means the total annual cost from that particular kind of infection is $270,000 dollars—the cost of one surgical infection multiplied by ten.

If the medical interventions include the use of newly acquired software, payment to staff and other materials, this adds up to $92,000. By proposing to spend that much, the hospital intends to have the surgical infections drop by half, thereby saving the hospital $135,000. This figure is derived by multiplying $27,000 by five—the cost of extended days avoided.

The benefit for the hospital in one year in this respect is $43,000 after $92,000 is subtracted from $135,000.

If the interventions do not result in any benefit whatsoever, with surgical infections continuing to increase, the hospital will need to carry out evaluations of a different kind to find out where the glitch is in the process. It could be that nurses or their assistants require more training in handling surgical patients, or perhaps there is a process failure that can be handled administratively.

Methods of Reimbursement

There are different methods through which institutions can reimburse the cost of health-care services. These include use of payer-based systems, P4P, payment bundling and purchase that is based on value.

Payer Systems

One category of payer system is self-pay, meaning that patients pay their medical bills directly, without any discounts. Another type of payer system involves pro bono work, where an institution does not charge a patient who cannot pay for treatment.

Another payer system is health maintenance organizations (HMOs). In this system, recipients of health care are required to pay a set fee for a comprehensive package of services; the basis of such payment is termed "capitation."

Then there is the prospective payment system (PPS). The payment here is made as per the patient type.

There is also the preferred provider organization (PPO), and within this payer type, patients pay for services as members of a group with negotiated rates. PPOs require that you select your physician of choice from a list of recommended ones, viewed as a network, so as to maintain costs at the negotiated level.

Point-of-Service-Organization (PSO) is another of the payer system types, and here recipients of health-care services also benefit from relatively low rates when they use providers who are members of a network. Those who prefer to use providers outside that network must pay higher rates.

Medicaid or Medicare is the last of the payer system categories, and it provides a range of options for making payments. Among them are HMOs, P4P, PPOs and prospective payments.

P4P Programs

Pay-for-performance (P4P) comprises programs that incentivize health-care institutions in order to encourage them to enhance the quality of their services. P4P comprises four features: performance, outcome, patient satisfaction and technology or structure.

Still, there are some P4Ps whose major interest is the reduction of costs. The incentives they give can be exemplified by rewarding doctors who prescribe fewer tests or who prescribe tests that are comparatively lower-cost but which are still helpful to patients.

Payment Bundling

Under this reimbursement method, several health-care providers are reimbursed via a single payment, rather than separately. This means the reimbursement is done for the services purchased by a patient rather than the cost incurred by individual health-care providers. One method of bundled payment initiated by the CMS Innovation Center, meant to enhance patient care at reasonable costs, is referred to as the Bundled Payments for Care Improvement Initiative.

Bundling of payments comes in four models, Model 1 – 4, with Medicare paying discounted rates in Model 1 on the basis of IPPS. In Model 2, payments are made for services rendered, and thereafter reconciliation of such payments is done by CMS against the anticipated costs. Any excess revenue is paid.

Model 3 is similar to Model 2, with the variation being that in Model 3, the focus is on the services that follow post-acute health care, which include SNF, HHA and care provided in rehabilitation centers. The period covered begins within a span of thirty days after the patient has been discharged, and it should not exceed ninety days.

The focus of Model 4 is the period of hospitalization for acute care; this is the purpose of prospective bundled payment.

Basing Purchasing on Value

Value-based purchasing is a program designed by CMS to be an incentive to hospitals that provide acute care. Such hospitals are expected to show that the care they provide to patients is of high quality. In addition to the payments made based on the fees charged, these hospitals receive extra payments as incentives.

When assessing quality, the process patients must undergo is taken into account, and to this end, certain measuring tools have been devised to measure quality in different situations or units. For example, if it is necessary for a patient to receive fibrinolytic therapy, it should be given within half an hour of the patient's arrival at the hospital.

The threshold given to hospitals is 50 percent, while the benchmark used is the average of the topmost decile. If a hospital's service improves to the extent of matching the given benchmark or exceeding it, the score given is nine. If performance falls below the given threshold, the score given is zero. And if performance lies between the threshold given and the benchmark, the score is picked from zero to nine.

Also, in a bid to ensure payments made match the value of services provided, a score is awarded for consistency. If consistency is measured above the benchmark, a score of twenty points is accorded to the hospital. Here also, any institution whose consistency in providing quality health care falls below the threshold scores zero, while those whose measure of consistency falls between the threshold and the benchmark are given scores between zero and twenty. When an institution's scores are added up, the final score is the Total Performance Score (TPS).

Contractual Agreement

Agreements of a contractual nature pertain not only to vendors but also to suppliers of materials as well as staff. When it is time to choose a suitable vendor, it is important that you choose from a range of vendors who have served other institutions similar to yours.

Choosing a Vendor

For the product the institution wants, prospective vendors should provide you with the history of the version they have first. They also should provide information as to how often they upgrade their products, and how compatible their product is with the equipment or software currently in use at your institution. The vendor should also inform you as to whether the firm offers after-sales service or maintenance.

Only after you are well informed about the products, conditions and terms of purchase, can you be in a position to identify the best vendor to enter into a contractual agreement with your institution. Besides information received directly from the vendors, you should do research online and make informal consultations with some of the institutions with whom you network. If there is a conference where the product you are interested in is going to be discussed, it is a good idea to attend because you can learn facts about the product and ask helpful questions of experts.

If you want to use a Request for Proposal (RFP), you can do so. An RFP's main purpose is to explain what the organization requires. Still, many vendors send standard responses to such requests, as opposed to submitting a customized response for each RFP. It is crucial to seek legal advice before finalizing a contractual agreement with a vendor, usually after it has been reviewed by the team, the institution has chosen to evaluate such contracts.

Among the important features to be included in a contract are terms of delivery as well as installation, staff training and support in the use of the product, liabilities, price, terms of payment, modification of programs and confidentiality.

Sourcing of Materials

When considering where to source material from, consideration should be given to minimizing cost. Most hospitals do their sourcing through Group Purchasing Organizations (GPOs), whose aggregating of purchase orders enables them to make their purchases in bulk, and that lowers costs of the materials and, by extension, helps the institution save money. Use of GPOs has been found to lead to savings within the range of 10 to 15 percent.

Although negotiation of contracts is done by GPOs, the actual buying of materials is done by the respective health institutions. Making hospital purchases through a GPO frees up staff that would otherwise have been needed to carry out the entire purchase process. Since that means a savings on working hours, the ultimate result is a savings on staff costs.

Other methods that health organizations use to try to keep costs down when sourcing materials is by dealing with just a few vendors and keeping the number of branded items to a minimum.

Staff Contracts

When members of staff are on contract, it means they have been engaged to work for a defined short period. A staff contract can be as short as a day. Many hospitals that hire staff on contract go through employment agencies; for some, this becomes necessary when they are short of staff.

Nevertheless, there are also instances where contract employees are engaged directly by a hospital, often to work on a particular project either for a short period or for a long duration.

Other staff members are referred to as "traveler workers," and even these have formal agreements with the health-care institution employing them. Doctors, nurses and therapists can belong to the category of traveler workers who are professionals under the employ of agencies that offer them attractive remuneration packages in order for them to make themselves available to work in different localities.

Although traveler staff members normally work in a station for a short period lasting four to twelve weeks, some contracts can last up to two years. Many of the agencies that have traveler nurses prefer RNs who have at least a year or two of practical experience, if not more.

These nurses are not only deployed within the state where they joined the agency; they can also be deployed to different states to offer health-care services. When this happens, a nurse is sometimes required to get licensed by her/his new state of residence, unless there is a Nurse Licensure Compact between the two states. Thirty-four states have an NLC in common, which means any nurse licensed in one of those states can work in another of these states without the need to be relicensed. It is worth noting that travel employees cannot be counted among the hospital staff for purposes of receiving benefits as they receive their remuneration from their respective agencies. Hospitals pay the salaries for the travel workers to the individual agencies.

Staffing Principles

Principles of staffing deal with issues pertaining to the positions given to employees as per their qualifications, employees' manner and level of remuneration and other matters that make staff feel well compensated and appreciated.

Full-Time Equivalent

Full-time equivalent (FTE) is sometimes referred to as whole-time equivalent (WTE). It is a measure of an employee's workload when the hours he/she works are divided by the official workweek's hours. Take, for example, an employee whose hours as per the duty schedule total forty. If the institution has a policy of a forty-hour week for staff, it means the FTE for this particular employee is: 40 hours ÷ 40 hours = 1.0.

One of the uses of FTE is serving as a measure of cost-effectiveness, especially when reviewing various levels of staff. In this regard, FTE is a favorite not only for employing institutions but also for agencies whose role is accreditation. The official FTE hours are 2,080 in a year, a figure arrived at after multiplying the weekly forty by fifty-two weeks.

If you are asked to calculate the number of FTE employees, you need to add up the hours all the employees have worked, and then divide the total by 2,080. If there are seasonal employees, do not include them in the determination of FTE. This is because seasonal employees are on duty for a period not exceeding 120 hours in a year. When calculating the FTE for a single employee, take 2,080 hours as the maximum number of hours worked, even if the actual number of hours the individual was on duty in the year exceeded that total.

Example of FTE Calculation

Calculate the FTE for 10 employees of ABC Hospital, whose actual hours worked include 2,340 for one employee, 2,080 for each of four employees, 1,040 for each of four other employees and 800 hours for the remaining employee.

Employees with 2,080 hours are 5 (1 + 4) = 2,080 x 5 = 10,400

Employees with 1,040 hours are 4 = 1,040 x 4 = 4,160

Employee with 800 hours is 1 = 800 x 1= 800

Total hours worked by all the employees = 10,400 + 4,160 + 800 = 15,360

FTE is therefore 15,360 ÷ 2,080 = 7.3846

Note that FTE is not given in numbers with decimal points; instead, such numbers are rounded down to the closest whole number. For that reason, the number of FTE employees the institution has is seven.

It is also worth noting that any employee whose workweek consists of thirty-six hours is considered a 0.9 FTE.

Hours per Patient Days

The term "hours per patient" is used in reference to the total number of hours one patient requires to be attended to by a health-care provider every single day on average. One of the ways to find this is by considering the entire patient population in the hospital. This gives you the average patient census. The patient census taken at midnight is preferred for use in this regard, and past and prevailing trends are also factored in.

Another important statistic is "nursing hours per patient day" (NHPPD). This considers the actual number of hours a given nurse is present to render patient care services. In short, a nurse's sick days must be excluded from this calculation.

Example of NHPPD Calculation

Average number of patients in Unit A = 20

Total nurses working in a day (in shifts) = 14

Average number of hours per nurse = 8

Total number of hours worked per day = 14 x 8 = 112

To find the NHPPD, divide the total period of productive working hours by the number of patients attended to. In this case: 112 hours ÷ 20 patients = 5.6 NHPPD

When calculating NHPPD, it is important to be precise on the hours that are effectively productive. There could be a nurse who, because of her/his benefits package, only works 80 percent of the normal 2,080 hours in a week, but gets paid 100 percent of the normal hours and is considered FTE. For purposes of calculating NHPPD, the productive hours utilized should be 80 percent of 2,080 hours—this means 1,664 hours are the total productive hours for this nurse.

How to Develop a Budget

Before learning to develop a budget, it is important to understand the major types of budgets used in the health-care industry: the operating budget, capital budget, cash budget and master budget.

The Operating Budget

The operating budget addresses the day-to-day needs of the institution, such as staff salaries, insurance, depreciation and general expenses, and also factors in profit. The three main features of the operating budget are revenue, expenses and statistics.

The budgets submitted by departments are usually of an operational nature. However, there may be variations in the approaches used by departments in different hospitals. The main approaches hospital departments follow in preparing their budgets include the fixed or forecast approach; the flexible approach; zero-based approach; responsibility center approach; the program approach; appropriations approach and the continuous or rolling approach.

In the fixed approach, budgetary items always remain the same, as a forecast is made of the expenses as well as revenue for the year under consideration. In the flexible approach, anticipated costs and revenue are incorporated as estimates, and the fixed costs are indicated separately from those of a variable nature. When the approach used is zero-based, every cost center is reevaluated every time a new budget is prepared. The purpose of such reevaluation is to decide if there are some cost centers that need to be eliminated, have their funding reduced or continue unaltered.

In the responsibility center approach, focus is on any department or unit of the hospital that has a single person in a position of general responsibility. Such a one-person unit is treated as a distinct cost center. The program approach deals with the budget in terms of the programs run by the institution. Those, plus the costs to be incurred, form the budget items alongside the anticipated revenue.

The appropriations approach simply means that in order to run the budget, requests for funding are made to the government, and when the money is received, it is duly appropriated. The rolling approach is where updates on performance against the budget are periodically made within the financial period, so that by the time of the next budget, all departments are aware and realistic about their spending, output in terms of volume and revenue.

The Capital Budget

The capital budget addresses long-term needs, which require expenditures of a capital nature like purchasing of modern machinery and building renovations. The expenses included in the budget are those to be incurred within the year, even though the assets bought are meant to last for several years. It should be remembered that the decision to incorporate a capital expense into the year's budget is only done after completion of a cost-benefit analysis and needs prioritization.

Capital expenditures must tally with the institution's strategic plan, which ordinarily reflects the goals of the institution for a span of five years. Such a plan always contains expenditures of a capital nature, both those approved and those proposed. Any expenditure on land, vehicles, systems of information technology, refurbishing of buildings and other assets that last for years is considered capital in nature.

The strategic plan, as a budget guide, should reflect the costs over the duration as projected, and also indicate where the funding is expected to be sourced.

The Cash Budget

The cash budget addresses the movement of cash within the year, factoring in the cash spent, including capital assets, and also cash received, whether as direct payment by patients or through reimbursements. This should be viewed as a cash flow, which shows if the institution is well prepared to pay for anticipated expenses.

The Master Budget

The master budget is a comprehensive budget that incorporates all the items in the operating, capital and cash budgets. If the institution has additional budgets such as ones specific to a particular region or specialization, these should also be incorporated into the master budget.

Variances in the Budget

Since a budget is a projection, it is not a surprise that the actual expenditures for individual budget items sometimes vary from the budget, as does revenue.

It is, therefore, recommended that costs of items, like labor, insurance costs and others forecast in the budget, be compared with the actual costs incurred in order to establish if the institution spent more or less on the items. Variances should be sought for both the operational and capital budgets. If the variance is positive, "F" is used to denote that fact, while if the variance is negative, either of the letters "U" and "A" are used. The items focused on when calculating variances are mainly labor costs, expenditure on materials, overhead costs and sales.

Components of Budget Variances

When preparing budget variances, analyses of different kinds are carried out. These include the net present value (NPV), analysis of throughput, discounted cash flow (DCF), payback and internal rate of return (IRR).

NPV is the variance between total inflow and total outflow.

Throughput analysis is used as a measure of a project's capacity to raise throughput by minimizing bottlenecks within the institution's systems.

DCF is meant to evaluate starting costs as well as those incurred on a continual basis; the same evaluation is performed for revenues. Future cash flow is estimated and then discounted appropriately to reflect the value in current times.

Payback analysis is done for the purpose of determining approximately how much it will take to have projects recoup the costs incurred in establishing and running them. In this assessment, a comparison is made between the starting cost and average annual revenue.

IRR is the real return on investment as a percentage. In the health sector, it helps to assess what cash flow looks like.

Note that NPV and IRR are available in Excel. There is a space to insert the initial cost of your given investment, and since this is a figure you already have on hand, you just need to insert it as a negative value.

Reducing Costs through Outsourcing

Health institutions often outsource some services or enter into contractual agreements with firms in a bid to reduce costs.

Many of these outsourced services pertain to something other than health care provided directly to patients, such as catering and housekeeping. Some health institutions also prefer to outsource their IT-related services as opposed to buying equipment, setting it up, training staff and paying for long-term maintenance.

There are also some areas where direct health-care services are outsourced. Among others, these include anesthesiologists, physicians who attend to departmental emergencies, imaging services and dialysis.

The most prevalent trend is to source these health-care providers from the agencies with which they have registered, and the institution therefore does not have to deal with payments directly. Considering the outsourced health-care providers do not work for long in one station, they are not hired for jobs that require them to establish long-term relationships with patients. In other words, it is unlikely for a hospital to hire a physician for the purpose of providing primary health care to patients.

How to Determine Optimal Workload

The workload staff has to shoulder depends on a range of issues like staff numbers at the hospital, patient population, NHPPD, unit type and patients' acuity levels. Acuity means the level of care an individual patient needs.

How Nurse-Patient Ratio Affects Workload

When some or all of the previously mentioned factors vary, the ratio of nurses to patients also varies. Sometimes one hospital can have a nurse-to-patient ratio of one to one in its intensive care unit, but that ratio might be one to five in the unit of general medical surgery.

How Skill-Mix Affects Workload

The nurse-to-patient ratio is also affected by the hospital's skill mix, and consequently, the staff workload is affected too. The effect skill mix has on workload can be seen in situations where one hospital only has RNs, and another only has licensed vocational nurses (LVNs), working alongside unlicensed assistive personnel (UAPs), under the supervision of RNs. The latter scenario results in a lighter workload because the RNs have staff to delegate some tasks to, leaving the RNs to handle the tasks that require specialized skills.

How Staffing Affects Workload

Sometimes the acuity of patients in a given unit is considered when determining the number of nurses to post to the unit. To be able to compare acuity among different patients, each person is allocated a score, and the factors influencing the scores are varied. They include the patient's diagnosis, how complicated his/her condition is and how complex the care he/she requires is. Often hospitals use computer-based programs to calculate the scores that reflect acuity.

The higher the score, the more intense the nursing care a patient requires. Some units need several float nurses, who are ready to be referred to any unit at a moment's notice.

Concepts, Styles & Principles of Leadership

For service delivery to be efficient, leadership must be effective. In this regard, it is crucial that the work environment be healthy, that the best leadership principles are followed and that the leadership understands the most applicable theories of management.

Leadership can be pervasive, servant type, situational or appreciative.

Pervasive Leadership

Leadership that is pervasive revolves around the notion that every individual has the potential to lead or influence other people. That is why, under this leadership, groups are given great autonomy in making decisions, as opposed to waiting for directions from a central leadership point.

Because of the belief in the capacity of every individual, employees are provided with the tools necessary to enhance performance, including training, mentoring and access to role models.

Servant Leadership

These kinds of leaders view themselves primarily as servants. They pay attention when their juniors have something to say, and they empathize with them. When they want something done, they use persuasion, and they encourage people to work with one another and to be significant participants in the things taking place in the organization.

Situational Leadership

Leadership is termed situational when it is flexible and able to adapt as situations change. One behavior typical of a situational leader is having the tendency to tell rather than discuss, meaning communication is one-way.

Another type of behavior is "selling." Unlike telling behavior, in this case, the situational leader's communication is two-way. These leaders are ready to offer support, both emotionally and socially.

Situational leaders also exhibit "participating" behavior. In this case, the situational leader identifies tasks that can benefit from participatory decision-making and gets all people involved.

The fourth type of behavior is "delegating," where the situational leader leaves task performance to the people he/she leads.

A great situational leader must have the capacity to diagnose needs and to correctly assess the individuals involved. This helps to determine the level of supervision necessary and how ready individuals are to learn.

Situational leaders must be adaptable, changing behavior as the situation requires. They must be able to communicate effectively, altering communication styles as necessary to get the message across.

Appreciative Inquiry

In appreciative inquiry, there is a presumption that every individual and every organization has something positive. This tendency to seek the positive relies on five important principles: constructionist, simultaneity, poetic, anticipatory and positivity.

Coaching

Leadership involves coaching, providing general career-related information and addressing issues that may be of concern. Nurse executives should be confident of their capacity to assert themselves and to be direct in confronting issues for the sake of resolving conflicts and promoting collaboration among staff members.

Mentoring

The most common mentoring model involves a mentor volunteering expertise while the mentee utilizes it. The major steps in the mentor-mentee relationship include

- selection of a mentor
- determination of expectations
- development of competency
- and the stage where the mentor leaves the mentee to practice independently, only offering advice when consulted.

Precepting

The nurse executive can act as a preceptor for those studying to become nurse executives, or to junior staff members at the health institution. A preceptor is simply a role model and the person someone goes to for guidance and consultation. It is important that a nurse executive be able to carry out clinical supervision as his/her normal role requires, even while guiding others.

Emotional Intelligence

The concept of emotional intelligence used in nursing was developed by Salovey and Mayer, and it means an individual's capacity to comprehend and manage personal emotions, along with the emotions of others.

This capacity is categorized into the capacity to perceive emotions, use them, understand them and manage them.

Howard Gardner's theory of multiple intelligence categories intelligence into seven types: linguistic, logical, visuospatial, kinesthetic, rhythmic, interpersonal and intrapersonal.

Nurse executives need to study the trait model and the Goleman & SEL emotional intelligence concept as well. They also should learn where influence and power come from. They must learn about self-reflection, how to evaluate one's own leadership, how integration of diversity is best accomplished and how to be sensitive in the workplace.

Change-Management Functions

It is crucial that nurse executives know how best to manage change so that normal activities at their institution are not disrupted and people affected do not feel disoriented. Proper change management involves five fundamental functions, which include:

Making a plan

1. Organizing resources and determining how to go about the changes
2. Implementing the changes and making any necessary adjustments along the way
3. Assessing the impact of the changes on a continued basis
4. Seeking feedback.

How to Make Relationships Effective

Once an individual has established relationships for the sake of change management, it is important to ensure those relationships are effective. Some characteristics needed in order to enhance effective relationships include sincere listening, having a positive presence as a leader and being a good communicator.

For a nurse executive to manifest positive leadership presence, it is imperative that he/she endeavors to remain friendly at all times and has a positive attitude. Other behaviors include being an active listener, sharing credit, providing feedback, engaging in conversations with staff and being prompt when solving problems.

Effective communication has some important aspects, one of them being the process, which should involve both verbal and nonverbal interactions. One should be able to read communication when it is delivered in a symbolic manner and be able to use symbolic language appropriately. It is also important to understand that communication is receiver-based, meaning it can only be effective if the recipient understands the intended message.

When communicating, nurse executives should also be conscious of the irreversibility of what has been uttered, and the unrepeatability of the original message. The latter underscores the importance of communicating effectively in the first instance because it is impossible to communicate the exact same thing a second time in the exact same way. The first time a message is communicated also has the strongest impact.

Other issues nurse executives need to familiarize themselves with include networking, creating a succession plan and how to make the environment conducive for interactions with employees.

Chapter 7: Health Care Delivery – Knowledge

This chapter addresses ethics that nurse executives should know and effect in the course of duty; business ethics; code of ethics as per the ANA; patients' advocacy; staff advocacy and advocacy for the nursing profession; standards of practice; and technological integration.

Principles of Ethics

Among the principles of ethics are those that focus on autonomy as well as justice, where autonomy means people have a right to make up their mind on how they want to receive care. Parents are legally responsible for making such decisions for their children.

Ethics holds that the scarce resources available within the health-care sector should be used fairly so that everyone in society benefits.

Health care also involves principles of beneficence and nonmaleficence, with beneficence involving doing things so that someone else benefits. It is the principle nurse executives and other health-care personnel are expected to follow as they treat patients and carry out other responsibilities.

The principle of nonmaleficence involves health-care providers not doing anything that is likely to harm a patient. This means that whatever action one takes should be both good and neutral in the moral sense. The doer's intention must also be good. The principle clarifies that one cannot take a bad action and anticipate good results.

Nurse executives should know how to facilitate decision-making, and one way to do so is to have an ethical framework. Nurse executives should be able to identify ethical frameworks, identify an issue that needs to be addressed, be clear about personal values and those of others and address any existing conflicts between the two. They should also be able to identify possible influencing factors and barriers, such as religion, regulations, medical status and socioeconomic situation. Nurse executives should be aware of how important veracity and confidentiality of information is.

Bioethics is another area nurse executives are expected to be conversant with. Bioethics follows the reasoning that among all the choices a medical practitioner can make involving caring for a patient, the path chosen must be the most correct from a moral standpoint.

Environmental ethics is a crucial area too, and it focuses on the assumption that every person has an ethical duty to the entire environment that encompasses all living beings. Health-care providers are thus required to protect the environment. Nurse executives should familiarize themselves with the different ways their institutions can help with environmental protection, one of them being recycling.

It is important that nurse executives learn about the decision-making model designed by Chally and Loriz in 1998, and how to deal with any ethical dilemma.

Business Ethics

In order to understand business ethics well, it is important to learn about corporate compliance, including the Privacy Act of 1974.

Programs relating to corporate compliance are initiated by the federal government through the Office of the Inspector General. However, every health-care institution is required to develop its own plan of compliance. The Affordable Care Act has mandated this from institutions that receive reimbursement from the CMS.

The 1974 Privacy Act restricts the kind of employee information a federal agency can gather and store in people's files. However, nongovernmental organizations can collect a lot more information and retain it, as they are not subject to federal restrictions like these. Still, it is possible to find states that have put legislation in place so that restrictions on possession of people's information covers even nongovernmental organizations. Federal law and some state laws also grant individuals the right to access their personnel files and letters of reference.

Code of Ethics as per ANA

The ANA developed the code of ethics for nurses, which has nine provisions.

1. Nurses must treat everyone with respect and consideration, their social standing notwithstanding.
2. A nurse must commit fully to a patient, any conflicts notwithstanding.
3. A nurse is required to promote and advocate for the health and safety of patients.
4. Nurses must maintain patients' privacy and confidentiality while at the same time, offering protection against any adverse practices.
5. A nurse is responsible for all practices carried out, including any delegated tasks.
6. A nurse should be exercise self-respect, maintain integrity and be competent.
7. A nurse must contribute to making the environment conducive to the provision of appropriate health care, as is professionally and ethically required.
8. Nurses must engage in the development of knowledge for the purpose of advancing the profession.
9. Nurses should collaborate with other health-care providers in their efforts to meet the needs of patients.

Nurses must be able to articulate the values of the profession and also promote and maintain its integrity.

How to Advocate for Patients

In order to adequately advocate for patients, nurse executives and other health-care providers need to acquaint themselves with the Patients' Bill of Rights. They should know what rights patients have, as reflected in the standards set by the Joint Commission and National Committee for Quality Assurance.

Patients' Fundamental Rights

It is the patient's right to be respected, to receive a response when in need and to decide the kind of care to accept. Other rights include access to means of airing grievances, privacy and confidentiality, safety from neglect or any form of abuse and protection when acting as a research subject.

A patient also has a right to have results appraised and to have access to information pertaining to the health institution, health practitioners treating him/her and the services being offered. Other rights involve procedures for appealing against decisions made pertaining to health-care services and/or an organization's ethical conduct and procedures pertaining to organ donation and procurement.

Other issues nurse executives should be conversant with include patients' access to quality health care, taking into account the costs involved, insurance coverage and physical location.

Nurse executives should also be knowledgeable in matters related to the safety of patients. They should be familiar with MedWatch and the 1990 Safe Medical Practices Act, which requires that any defective medical items be reported.

How to Advocate for Staff

As administrators, nurse executives should know how to advocate for their staff. They should ensure the work environment is healthy, make sure staff is treated fairly, provide the right equipment for staff to be able to render services and manage employees appropriately, including housekeeping and office staff.

Advocacy for the Profession

In order to advance the cause of nursing as a profession, nurse executives need to join professional bodies like the American Organization of Nurse Executives and the ANA. These platforms allow nurses to lobby for helpful policies.

Nurse executives must network expansively and consistently learn more about matters of significance that affect the practice.

Another way of advocating for the profession is to promote nurse education. Such advocacy is possible when staff has flexible work schedules, they are given incentives or rewards and they are accorded continuing education. There is also room for nurse executives to liaise with tertiary institutions to design relevant classes for their staff, such as an online BSN-bridging program.

Other factors that help enhance the profession involve lifelong education, being versed with the various professional certifications and supporting both certification and credentialing.

The Nurse Practice Act and Nursing Practice Standards

There is a Nurse Practice Act in every US state, along with a nursing board charged with its administration. In this document, one can find information pertaining to licensure and certification. The act also serves as the best reference point in matters regarding delineation of the scope of nurse practices, inclusive of the duties performed and the issue of delegation.

The act stipulates prerequisites for licensing foreign-trained nurses. The act also spells out the manner in which disciplinary issues should be handled.

The NCSBN Model Act

Nursing boards are guided in their role by the National Council of State Boards of Nursing (NCSBN). This act, together with the 2012 Rules & Regulations that were updated in 2014, provides the model that respective nursing boards should follow. The model is reflective of the most up-to-date practices, and the respective scopes of RNs, LPNs or LVNs, APRNs and UAPs are outlined.

Nursing Practice Standards

To understand the standards of nursing practice, one must be familiar with the guidelines of clinical practice, clinical pathways and also the American Nurses Association's scope and practice standards.

Clinical practice pathways, which relate to orders of medicines and protocols on antibiotics, are based on evidence. Under these guidelines, which have been developed or designed for use in several disciplines, are care plans that are specific to diagnosis, procedures and conditions. The pathways provide steps to be followed when providing care, along with the expected outcomes, and are used in standardizing care and reducing the length of patients' hospitalization. Each care plan needs to be documented, clearly showing the dates, applicable signatures, steps taken and outcomes observed.

It is important that a pathway be chosen on the basis of best practices, and its effectiveness must be continually monitored in order to determine if there are any modifications required.

Under the ANA scope and standards of practice is the 2015 Nursing: Scope and Standards of Practice as well as the Code of Ethics for Nurses.

When considering the practice scope, one should address who, what, when, how, where and why. As for the practice standards, one should address the duties and competencies every nurse is expected to carry out. There are seventeen nursing standards, the first six addressing the process of nursing, and the remainder addressing nurses' performance from a professional angle.

Regulatory and Compliance Standards

Legal matters include fraud, whistleblowing, compliance by organizations, HIPAA and a few more related subtopics.

Fraud

Fraud refers to the act of misrepresenting information for personal benefit. Another term used often used alongside fraud is abuse, which means behavior whose standard is below par and results in a fraudulently processed transaction such as rendering a service that is not medically necessary.

Different types of fraud include theft of medical identification. This form of fraud can be in the form of someone misusing someone else's medical identification number so as to receive health-care services or medical supplies, or it might involve the theft of a physician's identifier in order to illegally receive prescriptions or medical supplies.

Fraud can also be perpetrated when billing for medical items a hospital does not need; billing for items a hospital has not allocated funds for in the budget; upcoding of either materials or hospital services so that their reimbursement is calculated at a higher rate than the true rate; unbundling, which means having items that are normally billed as a package billed individually, thus inflating the amount to be reimbursed; and receiving kickbacks for giving referrals to other health-care providers.

Protection of Whistleblowers

When a whistleblower, a person speaking up to warn of fraudulent activities, provides information to his/her supervisor or anyone else internally, or to the media or other external party, he/she is protected under federal law. States also have laws protecting whistleblowers. The protection of whistleblowers falls under the Office of the Whistleblower Protection Program, overseen by OSHA.

Compliance by Corporations

Corporate compliance of a health-care institution involves being compliant with all applicable state and federal laws, any regulations by government or state agencies and maintenance of both ethical and legal standards.

Issues that are considered significant in seeking corporate compliance of a hospital or any other health-care institution include privacy and security as per HIPAA and HITECH when audits are conducted.

Others involve standards of accountability where staff discipline and confidentiality are observed, and privacy policies are adhered to.

Regulatory matters are also significant. These include EEOC and ADA; CMS and CLIA; the Federal Wage Garnishment Law and OSHA; EMTLA and Anti-Kickback law; Fair Labor Standards Act; Stark Law and the Family & Medical Leave Act.

An institution is required to comply with retaining records pertaining to its policies and practices. It must also conduct interviews appropriately and properly screen prospective employees.

Vetting or doing due diligence of third parties with whom the institution wants to deal with, like vendors, is of concern. An institution must also educate its staff about compliance with regulations.

Other matters of compliance include risk assessments, internal and external compliance-related audits and lists of sanctions by the government that include narcotics.

Role of HIPAA in the Health-Care Industry

The Health Insurance Portability & Accountability Act (HIPAA) ensures patients' rights pertaining to their health status are protected. Before a nurse can reveal any information regarding a patient, the patient must give consent. Moreover, any information of a personal nature, such as current and past health conditions and treatments received, is considered protected health information (PHI). This information should not be leaked in any form, whether written, electronically or verbally.

The exception to this rule is people who have durable power of attorney for the patients like spouses and legal guardians. Another exception comprises the individuals caring for the patient, such as physicians. Even then, whenever a physician wishes to discuss personal health issues with the patient when others, including family members, are present, the physician must first seek the consent of the patient and only proceed if he/she is in concurrence.

CFR, Title 45, Part 164 of HIPAA, explains the rules of privacy and security. The rule on privacy spells out the need for institutions to put in place measures to ensure patients' information is limited to only the mandated individuals. The rule on security stipulates that institutions must ensure the systems that hold patients' information are secure and compliant with established standards. Security stipulations include encryption of patients' information and assigning unique identifiers to patients, among others.

The Law Against Harassment

As administrators, nurse executives are expected to be conversant with laws pertaining to harassment involving anyone at the institution. There are a number of statutes that help in curbing different forms of harassment, and they include Title VII of the Civil Rights Act of 1964, Title IX of the Education Amendments of 1972 and the Civil Rights Act of 1991. The same purpose is served by the EEOC, which was established in 1980.

Besides these federal statutes, different states have additional laws against harassment of staff, including prohibitions against any form of discrimination.

The Issue of Sexual Harassment

Harassment of a sexual nature includes verbal utterances that are not welcome by the person being addressed, such as persistently asking for a date when someone is not interested, or making unwelcome suggestive comments. Other behavior that falls under the umbrella of sexual harassment includes physically touching someone without their consent.

Nurse executives need to be aware that, statistically, physicians top the list of culprits of sexual harassment in the health-care sector, although there are also cases of sexual harassment perpetrated by supervisors, colleagues and patients.

The Issue of Malpractice

When a nurse is found to have been involved in malpractice, he/she may be sued as an individual or in the name of the group he/she is associated with. If a nurse sued for malpractice loses the case, the state's nursing board does not need to be notified of the matter, because the charge is normally of a civil nature.

However, if the charge is negligence, the state's nursing board is notified and may decide to investigate whether any disciplinary measures are required. Negligence includes things like a nurse failing to refer a patient for necessary treatment when required, misdiagnosing a patient, providing the wrong treatment and failing to provide a guardian or family members with sufficient or required information.

The nurse is liable once he/she establishes a duty to someone by examining a patient or having a casual discussion where professional advice is sought, including on the phone. In order to avoid culpability, a nurse must follow up to ensure the patient is receiving proper health care.

The Issue of Negligence

When a staff member is accused of negligence, it means he/she failed to provide care to the standard expected.

The major categories of negligence include conduct of a negligent nature, gross negligence, negligence that is considered contributory and comparative negligence. A nurse's conduct is considered negligent if he/she fails to provide care that is reasonable as per his/her expertise and established standards. A charge of negligence can also be brought if a nurse fails to render assistance or protect a patient.

A nurse is deemed to be grossly negligent if he/she willfully provides insufficient care, in disregard for someone else's safety.

Contributory negligence pertains to a situation where a person being given care does something that jeopardizes his/her own welfare, thereby contributing to worsening his/her health status.

Comparative negligence is invoked when there is a need to compare the extent to which medical personnel involved in the treatment of a patient can individually be accused of negligence.

The GINA

The 2009 Genetic Information Nondiscrimination Act (GINA), a statute under EEOC, stipulates that employers should not make decisions on whether to employ an individual on the basis of the person or the person's family's genetic test results.

How to Plan & Respond to Emergencies

In order to plan and respond to emergencies appropriately, different kinds of possible disasters—both internal and external—must be assessed. Every hospital needs to have a Hospital Emergency Incident Command System (HEICS) on which the disaster response plan is based.

Disasters can involve large numbers of casualties arriving, such as during a train wreck, an epidemic, a fire, situations in the hospital where it becomes necessary to evacuate people or situations where a hospital is dangerously understaffed.

Emergency plans should include:

- staff access to information pertaining to disasters and drills
- having a clear command chain in place
- triage protocols
- assessing the extent of damage to the facility, which is normally a role for a health institution's safety officer

- ensuring the emergency department has the capacity to attend to incoming casualties
- protocols to be followed in transferring patients
- staffing matters, including means of having individuals report to work on an emergency basis
- putting communication systems in place both internally and externally, including being able to keep in touch with EMS staff
- having relevant supplies on hand.

Chapter 8: Health Care Delivery – Skills

Patient Experience Management

Some of the main steps in managing patient experience can be listed as follows:

1) Offer easy ways to schedule appointments via the internet, phone or in-person scheduling
2) Be friendly and attentive.
3) Have any forms that patients need to fill available online
4) Make sure that the waiting room is clean and comfortable
5) Respond to feedback
6) Stay in touch with patients

Evaluation of Health-Care Delivery Outcomes

It is important to evaluate the outcomes of health-care delivery and to prioritize delivery of care according to the findings. Nurse executives need to understand this evaluation by learning the factors that fall under it, like the nursing-sensitive indicators first identified by the ANA in 1994.

Other factors that fall under health-care delivery outcome evaluation include Institute of Healthcare Improvement Bundles (IHI bundles), ORYX® indicators, national patient safety goals, Leapfrog, the health-care buyers consortium, the magnet recognition program and the core measures of national quality.

It is also important for nurse executives to be well versed with suitable techniques for continued performance enhancement. Nurse executives must plan suitable actions to address any identified quality issues.

Technological Integration (Telehealth and E-health)

The term “telehealth” is used in reference to the provision of health-care services to people who live some distance away from health-care facilities. In such situations, medical personnel may interview patients by holding video conferences during which the concerned patients are diagnosed, monitored and treated.

Data like patients' blood pressure and heart rate is transmitted using "store-and-forward" technology. Sometimes the information is transmitted under very specific conditions, such as when a patient develops tachycardia and a medical professional must examine the patient's ECG.

Telehealth is increasingly gaining popularity because the population of elderly individuals continues to rise, and telehealth serves as a preventative measure. Once the emergence of health conditions is preempted, the result is a reduction in the number of hospitalization cases, and by extension, a drop in hospitalization costs for individuals, families and communities.

The Role of E-health in Patient Care

The term "e-health" refers to the use of information technology (IT) when delivering patient care. E-health is mainly linked to internet use, although sometimes it merely means computer use.

E-health comprises EHRs; Computerized Provider Order Entry systems (CPOEs); Clinical Decision Support Systems (CDSS); mobile-based health-related applications; telehealth services and telemonitoring services; virtually delivered health-care services and networks that are integrated.

Predictive Analytics

Predictive analytics are used in computer programs to determine the needs of a healthcare organization. This method uses existing data to forecast demands of patients up to 120 days in advance. This is a great emerging tool that will potentially help to curtail burnout and reduce the long shifts of nurses. Predictive analytics will help manage staffing needs as workflow patterns emerge in the workplace.

Remote Monitoring

Due to the everchanging nature of the world and especially due to the pandemic, remote monitoring has become essential in today's world. This process involves monitoring patients via a computer screen or cameras while the nurse is located in another physical location. Although many aspects of interaction are limited, nurses can still monitor and document details of patients as needed. Remote monitoring has a negative impact on the effectiveness of communication but can be helpful if a patient is in quarantine.

Chapter 9: Legal Matters and Health Care Delivery

The topic of health and public policy covers a variety of issues, including those of a legal nature.

How to Assess, Address & Prevent Legal Matters

It is important to understand the means nurses and other members of management have of assessing, addressing and preventing challenges of a legal nature.

The main means include:

- organizational or institutional transparency
- monitoring of compliance
- reacting to unfavorable reports in a manner that is not punitive
- putting in place mechanisms through which problems can be reported
- providing education and training to staff
- providing good leadership (by the administration)
- having policies that do not tolerate violations of standard work practices, especially with regards to bullying, violent behavior and harassment of a sexual nature.

How to Handle HIPAA Breaches

HIPAA's rule pertaining to a breach of policies regarding health-related information states that individuals affected should be notified within sixty days of the breach occurring. If ten or more people affected are unreachable, the information pertaining to the breach must be displayed on the institution's website for a period of three months or ninety days. A toll-free telephone number must also be provided on the site, or relevant notice be published in newspapers or broadcast via television or other electronic media.

If five hundred or more are affected by the breach, they should be contacted directly, and notice should also be published in major media outlets that serve the states with affected individuals. This should be done within sixty days of the breach occurring.

Also within the same period, the secretary to Health & Human Services (HHS) should be alerted through electronic media. If the breach affected a number of people below five hundred in number, information pertaining to the breach should reach the secretary to HHS within sixty days following the end of the year when the breach happened.

How Corporate Compliance is Facilitated

The inspector general of the HHS is in charge of providing guidance with regard to corporate compliance. According to that office, not only should hospitals, hospices and other health-care institutions comply with HIPAA rules of privacy and security, but they also should ensure accuracy in CMS billing.

Security as per HITECH

The Health Information Technology for Economic and Clinical Health Act (HITECH) falls under ARRA, the 2009 American Recovery and Reinvestment Act. It requires that notification be made to individual persons as well as the HHS regarding security breaches of personal health information.

The act also provides that regulations pertaining to security of information must be adhered to, or those who flout the regulations will face stiff penalties. Furthermore, this act prohibits the selling of information regarding an individual's health. If a person's health information is disclosed without the individual's consent, the person affected must be notified.

In order to meet the stipulations of HITECH, health institutions are encouraged to install EHRs, and incentives are awarded toward this end. There is also a penalty against institutions that fail to make use of EHRs, in the form of reduced payments for Medicare, unless the institution has been exempted from such installations.

It is important to note that both HIPAA and HITECH require that data and information pertaining to people's health be encrypted if being transmitted via the web, for the sake of confidentiality and protection. Such encryption protects not only personal health information but also other personal information like addresses and phone numbers, dates of birth, social security numbers and credit card details.

Making Health Care Consumer-Driven

The issue pertaining to consumer-driven health care involves making formal reporting public and adhering to CHNA and HCAHPS, among other requirements.

What Public Reporting Entails

When health-care institutions' performances are evaluated, the results must be made public, even if it means putting it up on a bulletin board within the institution. This is federal law and is also state law in approximately twenty-five states.

Measures used in assessing the performance of health-care institutions have been provided by CMS and AHRQ. The Affordable Care Act also requires public notification of performance assessments.

Community Health Needs Assessment

A Community Health Needs Assessment (CHNA) involves assessment of the services provided by health-care institutions, with a view to determining what other services institutions need to make available.

The steps involved in this assessment of needs include:

- determining the demographics within a given community
- assessing how involved consumers of mental health services are
- assessing how readily available psychiatrists are, alongside agencies that provide mental health–related care
- affordability of mental health-care services
- how accessible areas that need the services are
- assessing the existence of barriers or challenges that make it difficult or impossible to provide health care, like not having insurance, language barriers, discrimination or a shortage of medical staff.

The Role of the HCAHPS

The Hospital Consumer Assessment of Healthcare Providers and Systems (HCAHPS) is a standardized survey that is used at the national level to seek the opinions of patients regarding the quality of care received in hospitals. This survey, designed by a consortium of HCAHPS in collaboration with the Agency for Health Research & Quality (AHRQ), contains thirty-two items. The US National Quality Forum has endorsed this survey.

Hospitals that operate under the Inpatient Prospective Payment System (IPPS) are expected to carry out surveys. In order for CMS to process their reimbursements, institutions must submit their data. Institutions not under the IPPS do not have this requirement.

HCAHPS is included in the Affordable Care Act as a crucial element to be taken into account when calculations are being done for the consideration of Value-Based Purchasing programs (VBPs). The patients surveyed must have been recently discharged. Although there is a set of standard questions for use in the surveys, individual hospitals are permitted to add their own questions specific to their areas of special interest.

The Relevance of Healthgrades

Healthgrades is a privately owned company in the US, which has taken upon itself to collect data regarding more than three million health-care providers. This information is not only about health-care institutions, but also about individual doctors and a host of other participants in the health-care sector.

The company ranks hospitals according to patient mortality and complication rates. It also ranks doctors according to the professional experience they have, the rate at which their patients develop complications and according to how patients feel about the care received.

Healthgrades sources its information through Medicare and additional sources. The company's website is structured so that interested parties can seek information per medical specialty, individual hospital and/or specific doctor.

Matters of Public Policy

It is crucial that nurse executives be conversant with prevailing matters relating to health and public policy, so as to be able to develop and respond appropriately to plans for the future. Nurse executives must continually update themselves via various resources like the websites of relevant government agencies, health journals, the CDC and health conferences.

It is also important that nurse executives review statistics pertaining to different demographics, new emergence of diseases and other statistical information that can help meet the needs of patients.

At the same time, nurse executives should consciously take an interest in what is happening beyond the US as far as health and other issues are concerned. In this regard, they should be able to identify regions with outbreaks of diseases like Ebola, avian flu or COVID-19, etc. When planning policies, matters of staffing need to be taken seriously, including addressing any nurse shortages the health institution might be facing. It is also advisable to consider how work conditions for staff can be made more flexible.

The Role of ACOs

Accountable Care Organizations (ACOS), established under the Affordable Care Act, are groups comprising doctors, hospitals and other health-care institutions, which partner on a voluntary basis for the sake of providing health care to Medicare patients.

ACOs' main aim is to enhance the quality of health-care services and reduce costs. ACO members work in coordination with one another, ensuring health-care services are not duplicated. ACO members share the savings made through such coordination, and the amount is distributed by Medicare. There are various types of ACOs.

Categories of ACOs

The types of ACOs include the shared savings program, advance payment model and the pioneer model. The shared savings program involves qualified, participating fee-for-service members being paid, while the model for advanced payment entails receiving payments up front on a monthly basis, for the purpose of investing in staff and infrastructure. The advanced payment model is considered supplementary to the shared savings program.

As for the pioneer model, it is available only to well-established health institutions, whose shared payments are higher than the other categories.

The Role of PCMHs

Patient-Centered Medical Homes (PCMHs) are programs through which patients are accorded care, with their very first contact being the primary-care physician. This doctor is responsible for coordinating the care given to the patient by different partners, including the patient's family members and different medical personnel.

Basic Features of a PCMH

All PCMHs are required to be accessible to patients seeking health-care services, and the services provided must be comprehensive. This means not only are acute-care services provided, but ailments of a chronic nature are also treated. Additionally, services like diagnostics, different therapies and disease prevention are provided.

Another characteristic of PCMHs includes ensuring effective health-care services by hiring physicians who are capable of handling the health challenges of the target demographic.

PCMH doctors are required to coordinate the care given to patients by various health-care providers, ensure teamwork and provide safe, high-quality care that is based on facts.

Clinics Led by Nurses

Clinics overseen by nurses mostly provide outpatient health-care services. The nurse in charge must be an advanced practice nurse (APNs) who has a postgraduate degree. Many clinics overseen by APNs focus on disease prevention and chronic ailment management.

Delivery of Inpatient Care

Delivery of health care to inpatients happens once a patient has been officially admitted to a health-care institution. Medicare & Medicaid reimbursements are provided for such admissions.

If a patient spends the night at the hospital under observation after being treated for an emergency, such a patient is still considered an outpatient. A hospital census is carried out on a twenty-four-hour basis, a period that starts at exactly 12:01 a.m.

It is acknowledged that patient census can vary in the course of one day, and for that reason, every hospital must designate a particular time when a patient census is consistently performed. Every patient who is counted at census time represents a single inpatient service day.

How to Calculate Rate of Bed Occupancy

Bed-count days are the total of inpatient beds available within a given period. In order to determine what the rate of bed occupancy in a given hospital is, the following formula is applied:

Bed Occupancy Rate (inpatient) = (No. of Inpatient Service Days for Period A ÷ No. of Bed-Count Days (inpatient) for Period A) x 100

Once a patient is discharged, his/her length of stay (LOS) is immediately calculated as it is of particular importance as far as Medicare reimbursement is concerned.

How Ambulatory Care Works

Ambulatory care means the health-care services provided to people as outpatients, as opposed to inpatients. Often such patients are treated at physicians' offices or in clinics, urgent care centers, surgery centers, dialysis centers or hospitals.

Reimbursement of expenses incurred receiving ambulatory services is handled in a different manner from services provided to inpatients. Also, these services normally cost less than inpatient services and are considered one way of cost-saving. Ambulatory services are broadly provided by medical personnel in private practice, or by staff under the employment of organizations that provide ambulatory care, a good example being HMOs.

A part of the health-care services provided to inpatients falls under ambulatory care, like the services rendered at the emergency room, services of a diagnostic or therapeutic nature like radiation and some surgeries.

Home-Based Health Care

Health-care services are deemed to be home-based when the personnel providing the care travel to the home of the patient. Services for patients who are homebound are provided on an intermittent basis. Intermittent implies fewer days than seven in one week, or fewer hours than eight in one day, for a period of twenty-one days or shorter, within a span of sixty days. This is considered one care episode.

It is important to note that if a type of care is provided by a skilled nursing facility, it can also be provided at home by an agency that specializes in home-based health care.

A patient who is identified as fit for home-based care is one that a doctor considers suitable to be safely treated away from the hospital. This is something that the doctor in charge of the patient needs to certify before home care is started.

Intermittent care services may include treatment via IV; counseling and nutrition-based therapy; services from social workers; occupational, speech therapy and physical therapy; case management and services involving supporting the patient and/or providing care of a personal nature.

Any patient with the original Medicare is fully reimbursed for home care and is only expected to make a payment of 20 percent as a proportion of the Medicare-approved expenses for medical facilities or equipment considered durable.

Rehabilitation Services

A rehabilitation center can be a part of a nursing facility, like a department, although there are centers that specialize solely in providing rehabilitation services. Rehabilitation center programs include treating patients with physical injuries and offering therapy to help patients recovering from a stroke, brain and cardiac issues, among others. For instance, an elderly patient being treated at the hospital for a hip injury may then receive physical therapy at a rehabilitation center.

Some rehabilitation services are comprehensive, like those that offer speech therapy and occupational therapy to their clients. Patients receiving services at rehabilitation centers can either be outpatients or inpatients, usually depending on the number of hours they need to receive therapy each day. Medicare, Medicaid and insurance generally cover rehabilitative therapies geared towards improving an individual's functionality or inhibiting more deterioration.

US SNFs

Skilled nursing facilities (SNFs) in the US provide an array of services meant to improve the health of their clients. Their services are not strictly medical, as they also provide personal care to the clients. This includes dressing patients and helping them perform day-to-day activities, feeding and bathing them.

Sometimes patients are taken to SNFs after being given acute treatment. Many such patients require a stay of between a few days to six weeks. In addition to the usual services, the SNFs can provide physical or occupational therapy; and if needed, respiratory therapy can be provided.

It is not unusual for patients to continue receiving treatment at SNFs till their death, some of them having long-term insurance, but not Medicare. For Medicaid at the state level to cover such patients, they must meet some age and medical condition stipulations, as well as stipulations based on level of income.

Other Home-Based Care Providers

Other institutions that provide health care away from conventional hospitals include residential care facilities, assisted living facilities and facilities providing respite care.

Acute & Subacute Care

Hospitals are the main institutions that provide acute care, with procedures in place to diagnose patients' medical issues like MRIs, CTs, X-rays and laboratory-based procedures.

Services provided in subacute facilities range between those offered in acute hospitals and SNFs and nurses who are skilled in full-time attendance. Patients requiring subacute services normally take up four to six hours each in a day, although they may also require intensive therapies.

Laws & Regulations

Nurse executives are expected to be conversant with the bodies in charge of regulating how services are delivered in the health-care sector and must ensure the pertinent laws and regulations are adhered to.

The health industry has government and state agencies that ensure proper structures of health-care delivery and that utmost care is provided by hospitals and other health-care institutions. The Joint Commission is also central in the regulation of service delivery.

The Joint Commission

Within the United States, the body charged with establishing the standards of accreditation for individual health-care delivery programs is the Joint Commission. In addition to setting the competency levels required for different levels of practitioners, it also issues national patient safety goals on an annual basis. For an institution to be accredited, its performance is evaluated, with great focus being put on the efficiency of its processes, where actual outcomes are taken into account, and issues pertaining to patient safety and care are assessed.

Surveyors working for the commission normally check documents to see if an institution qualifies for compliance validation. They also inspect and observe activity on-site, interview staff, review delivery standards and medical records, review systems providing support and check how well data for measuring performance is integrated.

Centers for Medicare & Medicaid Services

The Centers for Medicare & Medicaid Services manage Medical A & B at the federal level. Medicare A is insurance catering for acute treatment nursing and other health services that are based at home, as well as hospice services for those with terminal ailments.

Medicare B is insurance that covers doctors and CNSs as well as laboratory tests, physical therapy and occupational therapy. Medicare Part A has its own list of benefits, as does Medicare Part B, but in the latter, the patient does not need to file a Medicare claim. These two parts, A and B, are commonly referred to as the original Medicare.

Among the different Medicare programs are the PPS, PPO, pay-for-service, which is a privately funded Medicare plan insurance, and specialty plans.

As for Medicaid, which is a program meant to provide welfare to individuals, and which is under the management of both the federal and state government, it is also regulated by the Centers for Medicare & Medicaid Services. Its authorization is under Social Security's Title XIX. The target group for Medicaid comprises people in the low-income bracket, and the aim is to ensure they also have access to required health-care services.

Adults who are foreigners, legally in the US and benefit from Medicaid, can only continue benefitting from it for five years. It is important to note there are states that offer Medicaid for measures of prevention, in the form of programs based either in homes or communities.

Chapter 10: Nursing Practice Models and Staff Development

Services begin to have an interdisciplinary look when nurses work in collaboration with physicians, pharmacists and social workers. Other disciplines involved in enhancing the health-care environment include nutritionists and therapists of varied specializations such as physical therapists and occupational therapists.

The Massachusetts General Hospital Professional Practice Model

This model is patient-centered, with nine elements to ensure cohesiveness and effectiveness when interdisciplinary health-care services are provided. An RN is accountable for the standard of care a patient receives.

The nine elements are:

1. Patient-centeredness
2. Vision and values
3. Nursing practice standards
4. Narrative culture
5. Development of professional nursing
6. Clinical recognition and advancement of the nursing role
7. Decision-making collaboration
8. Research
9. Interdisciplinary teams.

Relationship-Based Care

Relationship-based care, otherwise referred to as Koloroutis, is a model of professional practice that focuses on three fundamental relationships the health provider has with patient and family, self and colleagues.

This model is meant to ensure there is effective communication among the closest stakeholders, so the results of the health-care services provided are the best possible for the patient. Openness in communication and respect among team members is strongly emphasized.

The Synergy Model

The synergy model, a development of ACCN, ensures that patients' needs are central to everything a nurse does. The model comprises eight characteristics of a patient and eight competencies of a nurse, with the evaluation of the competencies being done on a scale of one to five.

The eight characteristics of the patient are

1. Resiliency
2. Vulnerability
3. Stability
4. Availability of resources
5. Complexity
6. Participation in provision of care
7. Participation in decision-making
8. Predictability.

The eight competencies of nurses are

1. Clinical judgment
2. Advocacy
3. Practices of care
4. Collaboration
5. Systems thinking
6. Clinical injury
7. Responses to the issue of diversity
8. Learning facilitation.

The third element that is fundamental to this model is the environment within which the health-care system exists. This must support patients' needs and empower the nursing practice.

The Watson or Human Caring Model

The model, which has a holistic approach to health care, is named after Jean Watson, who developed it as a human caring philosophy in 1979.

This model encompasses ten caring methods or caritas, which include the manifestation of love, kindness, equanimity and showing creativity when providing care, among others.

The Peplau Model

This model, considered the nurses' model of interpersonal relations, was developed by Hildegard Peplau in 1952. Its focus is the interaction between the nurse and the patient, who is the client.

Peplau believed the entire environment comprising the social, psychosocial and physical aspects could affect a person's health either positively or negatively. She considered the nurse to be a "maturing force," one with the capacity to direct the way a patient views his/her illness, and one who can help the patient consider that illness a learning experience that can leave a patient more matured in life. Nurse-patient collaboration is given utmost importance in this regard.

Other models and theories nurse executives need to learn about include the 1959 Orem theory by Dorothea Orem, differentiated nursing practice, the Orlando theory developed by Jean Orlando and the Leininger theory by Madeleine Leininger.

Delineation of Roles

Delineation of roles involves credentialing as well as privileging, where credentialing represents the process through which an individual's credentials to provide care to patients are verified as per the bylaws of an organization. Bylaws can vary from one institution to another, so credentials that are acceptable in one institution will not necessarily be accepted in another one. Privileging is only granted after credentialing has been completed.

Normally, health-care institutions have a committee in place for the sake of making decisions pertaining to credentialing and privileging. Nevertheless, some institutions prefer to rely on web services for verification of credentials.

The credentialing committee determines the qualifications required for individual positions at the institution, and such decisions are made on the basis of a range of considerations, inclusive of professional standards and licensure, guidelines of a regulatory and accreditation nature and several others.

Bill of Rights for Nurses

The bill of rights for nurses under the ANA is not legally binding but provides a list of the rights nurse professionals qualify for. These should serve as the basis for creating policy.

Among those rights are:

- the right to fulfill obligations pertaining to the welfare of patients and society
- the right to carry out work within an environment conducive to adherence to professional standards, and also within a nurse's scope of duty
- the right to operate within an environment that is ethically healthy
- the right for nurses to be their own advocates and their patients' advocates without worry of possible retribution
- the right to be paid fairly as per a nurse's level of education, professional qualifications and experience
- the right to work within a safe environment
- and the right to participate in negotiations for remuneration either as an individual or as a group.

Development of Clinical Staff

The best way of developing clinical staff revolves around orientation, continuing education, evaluation of activities appropriate for credits in continuing education, validation of competency, peer review and planning.

Orientation

When planning to develop a staff orientation, the nursing specialist concerned should consult with administrators at the departmental level, so as to have relevant information and insight, and also as a show of respect for the positions they hold and the experience they have. Such consultations can help enhance cooperation going forward.

Orientation also involves assessment of needs and putting in place a program for mentoring staff, which is mainly meant to provide support for nurses in the course of their work, to accord them a chance to learn from the expertise of colleagues and seniors.

Continuing Education

Continuing education involves the education and training required for an individual to remain abreast of what is happening in the world of nursing. Every nurse requires continuing education to remain relevant, and in many cases, employable. Continuing education is a requirement for renewing one's licensure.

Some states assess continuing education in terms of units, where, for example, a nurse is accorded a single unit for every hour worked. There are states that require confirmation that a nurse has earned twenty to thirty such units within one period of licensing, mostly a period of two years.

Some states have additional conditions like a requirement that the individual takes a course on how to handle end-of-life or HIV cases.

Evaluation of Continuing Education Credits' Activities

For activities to qualify for continuing education credits, they must meet the ANCC's criteria. Among others, the criteria include addressing a gap within the nursing practice, being based on assessment of needs and being free of commercial interference or influence.

Validation of Competency

Validating competency starts with selecting suitable criteria for use. Requirements for certification and job description are some aspects that must be reviewed. Once the required competencies have been compiled, the scores should be given within a range of one to four or a similar suitable scale.

Peer Review

In peer review, a medical professional is reviewed by colleagues in an intensive process. One may be reviewed individually or as part of a group, with available data being used as the basis for analysis. Often peer review in health-care institutions is carried out within departments under the guidance of a committee, and the system of ranking used reflects one's adherence to set standards.

Planning

Planning that is done for the sake of developing clinical staff starts with an initial staff assessment. Existing skill mix, diversity, staff motivation and empowerment are considered. The nurse executive also takes into account the institution's needs as far as issues of staffing, staff education levels and patient data are concerned.

Creation of a Professional Environment

It is important that a professional environment be created that is favorable for decision-making by an empowered workforce. Some of the ways of creating such an environment include sharing of governance, use of partnership councils, embracing accountability and delegation, engaging in critical thinking and civility.

Governance Sharing

When departments or teams are allowed to make their own decisions, this is tantamount to being given room to share in governance. A good example is the development of a work schedule for the department.

Partnership Councils

Having partnership councils is a form of evolved shared governance, with councils comprising personnel from all disciplines within the institution. Since there is normally a council at every level, the heads represent the respective councils at the higher-level council—the central partnership council. The role of this higher council is advisory and has the chance to share the role of making decisions with the institution's administration.

Accountability & Delegation

One way of developing a professional environment is to have members of staff take responsibility at a personal level for what they do. Also, one must be conscious of the legal implications of carrying out specific actions, and keep in mind that when a task is delegated, accountability is not. It is important for staff to understand the right conditions for delegating work.

1. The task to be delegated must be right, keeping in mind that different individuals may be suited to carrying out different tasks.
2. The circumstances under which delegation is being done must also be appropriate. A member of staff might know how to do something, but carrying out the task when resources are inadequate or within time constraints may be too much for the same individual.
3. The individual you delegate a task to should be right, and this goes beyond the individual's willingness to do the job. You must establish that the education, skills and professional level of the individual make him/her suitable for the task.
4. It is crucial that the person to whom work is being delegated is informed of the expectations. This includes providing a task description, the expectations for it and the expected results.

Once a task is delegated, the person delegating should have a way of supervising it. That person must intervene as needed and assess the task upon its completion.

Critical Thinking

For critical thinking to be successful, a number of elements must be factored in, including skills, interpretation, analysis and evaluation, as well as inference, explanation and self-regulation.

Standards must also be taken into account in critical thinking. Some elements identified in the 2001 publication of Paul & Elder serve as standards necessary for critical thinking. They include:

- clarity of concepts
- accuracy of data and all information
- precision in the manner information is communicated
- relevance of data
- helpful depth of information
- reasonable breadth of information so a reader can understand it from different perspectives
- logical arguments
- significance of information
- fairness towards fresh ideas.

Important Steps in Solving a Problem

In order to be able to anticipate a problem or prevent a recurrence of a problem, a hypothesis is necessary. One also needs to do the required testing and assessment of data to determine if the hypothesis is reliable. This involves defining the challenge, collecting data, pinpointing crucial concepts, weighing the reasons for taking specified actions and finally, making a decision.

Civility

Civility, which means treating other people respectfully, is necessary for a healthy working environment. Administrators like nurse executives must swiftly address any instances of rude or inappropriate behavior.

In order to develop a culture of civility within an institution, an existing problem must be identified. This can be done by carrying out surveys.

Next, a clear code of conduct for the staff must be established, spelling out the expected behavior and manner of communication. It is a good idea to identify some actions that constitute bad behavior, such as hazing, being sarcastic and eye-rolling.

Training all staff on how best to communicate dissatisfaction is important. Finally, it is crucial that offending members of staff be warned or punished so that everyone can understand the institution has zero tolerance toward inappropriate behavior.

Staff Recruitment

Recruitment of staff can be a big challenge when there is a nationwide shortage of staff; for that reason, it is important to know the factors to prioritize recruitment.

Factors to Prioritize During Staff Recruitment

Quality should be given preference over all other factors, and that fact should be reflected in all job postings.

The institution should take orientation programs seriously, where newly recruited staff can be mentored and/or undergo special training or programs.

It is also recommended that health-care institutions establish relationships with nurse training schools, so that nurse trainees can get work experience. Nurse graduates have a tendency to seek employment in the hospitals or health-care institutions where they did part of their training because of their familiarity with the staff and the environment.

The administration should cultivate a culture where everyone at the institution is welcoming to new staff members.

Also, in order to reduce the problem of finding qualified staff, the institution should be willing to remunerate its staff competitively. Besides making the pay package attractive, providing benefits not only makes it easy to find qualified job applicants, but it keeps staff turnover low. Another factor to consider involves working hours. If these hours range from eight to twelve, and there is flexibility of the work schedule, nurses are more likely to find the hours favorable.

People want to work in an institution that gives them room to advance their education or training, and so it is worth considering supporting staff to develop their careers. They should be provided with facilities for continuing education, which is crucial for renewal of professional licenses. It is also helpful to have a program in place through which assistance can be given to staff members.

Staff Recognition

Institutions need to recognize staff members who have excelled in their work. This positive reinforcement does not have to be monetary; it can be in written form or be an announcement to other staff members, for example.

How to Retain Staff

When a hospital has too few nurses compared to the number of patients, the quality of care may be compromised. For that reason, it is important to know what to do in order to retain staff before contemplating recruiting new hires.

When staff retention is being considered, the potential for some staff members to retire in the near future should be taken into account. To retain staff, and also when hiring, make payment packages attractive, allow for flexible working hours, provide a supportive work environment, etc.

Internal Customer Service

Internal customer service is provided to people within the health-care institution, including coworkers. If the services provided internally are wanting, those services that the health-care institution provides externally can be adversely affected.

Customer service within the health-care institution involves ensuring staff has everything needed in order to carry out duties appropriately, including equipment. Furthermore, excellent internal customer service entails:

- respect for every member of staff
- having known standards of service delivery
- providing continuing education for all staff
- ensuring administrative personnel are available when members of staff need them
- and keeping communication channels open.

External Customer Service

Customer service is deemed external when health-care institution staff interacts with people from outside the institution. The external parties include patients, suppliers of medications and equipment, insurance firms and others.

Communication between the insiders and the outsiders needs to be clear, smooth and appropriate, whether it is carried out by phone, via email, face-to-face, etc.

Importance of Service Recovery

Service recovery refers to appeasing a dissatisfied customer. The presumption here is that such a person might not only be offended but that his/her trust in the institution could be drastically reduced, if not entirely lost.

A good example is a patient made to wait an hour longer than promised for minor surgery when an emergency case is brought into the hospital. An equally good example is a patient developing a serious infection following surgery. In both of these cases, the goodwill of the patients involved may be eroded.

The recommendation is that you immediately acknowledge the client is justifiably unhappy, and follow that with an apology. Health-care providers need to understand that there is a difference between apologizing and taking the blame for whatever upset the client. Acknowledging the client's feelings and offering an apology makes it easier to move forward with fruitful service delivery, as opposed to denying the issue, a situation that only exacerbates the client's resentment.

Nurse executives must create a vision that enhances care that puts family as the central focus. A good example is when a parent brings a child to the hospital. It is important that the physician and nurses involve the patient in a discussion pertaining to the course of treatment the health-care providers deem suitable.

When care is family-centered, there is frankness in communication between the staff and the patient's close family members or guardians, and parties on either side respect the other's opinion.

Chapter 11: Strategic Planning & Visioning

In this chapter, you will learn about the principles of planning strategically; how to develop a new program; the trends that affect nursing and health-care delivery; how to communicate, build consensus and get people to support the proposed strategic plan; how to measure performance; how to evaluate processes and results over a set period; the important features of a plan and how to manage a project.

The first principle involves alignment of the strategic nursing plan with the organizational or institutional plan, which should be done from the very start. Resources and management support are needed for any strategic plan to be implemented successfully. For instance, if the organization plans to raise productivity for the sake of reducing costs, the strategic nursing plan should include an initiative to reduce the ratio of nurses to patients. The result of a reduced nurse-patient ratio is a reduction of hours of overtime worked, which translates to a reduced labor expense.

SWOT Analysis

One of the important undertakings when implementing a strategic plan is a SWOT analysis, which means analyzing the strengths of the nursing function, its weaknesses, opportunities available and existing or impending threats.

All those factors should be considered both internally and externally. For example, the nursing function may be currently well funded, so from an internal point of view, that is a strength, which is accompanied by an internal weakness of a high wage bill. In the meantime, opportunities can be identified in a growing population, and there may be few threats to the nursing function coming from outside.

Organization's Strategic Plan

A strategic plan covers a long period, like ten to fifteen years. Factors that need consideration for the nursing strategic plan to succeed include strategic quality planning, assessing customer needs and satisfaction, creating a vision statement and mission statement and developing goals and objectives.

Development of a New Plan

When developing an entirely new plan, it is important to start by writing a proposal. Sometimes an inquiry letter is required first.

It is also important to prepare a proforma, a statement outlining anticipated expenditures in the proposed program. The proforma, normally a spreadsheet, reflects both revenue and expenses and covers an entire year or longer. Items appearing in a proforma include net revenues, all direct expenses like salaries and contribution margins and indirect expenses like overheads.

Features of a Business Plan

The important elements to include in a good business plan include:

- an executive summary
- a service or product description in brief
- management's structure or hierarchy
- a market survey
- a market strategy.

A good business plan must also detail organizational operations, like methods of controlling quality and inventory, a timeline, risk factors and an appendix.

Nurse executives are required to learn about marketing, especially related strategies, and must understand the target market.

Trends that Affect Nursing & Health-Care Delivery

One of the factors that affect nursing and service delivery is the environment within which nurse executives and other nurses operate. It's important to study trends so that they can be factored into nurse teaching programs and other's various activities.

Among the significant trends are the use of portable medical gadgets and robotic surgical equipment, social networking, use of IT alongside systems analyses, use of home-based care delivery and reduced periods of hospitalization, focusing on wellness and nutrition as well as preventative care, focusing on sustainability and recycling and providing personalized patient care.

Communication, Consensus Building & Strategic Plan Support

It is important for communication to begin even before a strategic plan is presented. Even if strategic plans are designed by the executive, implementing them in a successful manner requires input from all members of staff.

It is imperative that a nurse executive explain the outline of the strategic plan to all stakeholders, including department heads, emphasizing the plan's benefits. Eventually, when it is time to explicitly ask for support, it's appropriate for the nurse executive to mention any lingering concerns, and to let the other people know the concerns can be surmounted with their positive participation.

Measurement of Performance

In order to measure performance, a benchmark must be identified against which progress will be gauged. It is also important to note where the process stands at the current time. In short, there needs to be a baseline, which can be established by assessing the current state of affairs. For example, what was the monthly number of patients readmitted last year, on average?

It is also usual for nurse executives to use national or state data as a benchmark for a process. Some credible sources of data for benchmarking include Hospital Compare; AHRQ; Becker's Hospital Review; HEDIS; CMS and the National Committee for Quality Assurance.

Process Evaluation & Outcome Measurement

In order to evaluate the progress of a given project, current procedures must be measured and monitored. One of the most important aspects of such evaluations is identification of deviations because it provides an opportunity to make corrections early. Risks are also assessed and duly managed.

Important Features of a Project Plan

The important features of a project plan include:

1. Purpose

2. Scope
3. Plan requirements
4. A schedule of all activities
5. Finances
6. Quality control
7. Resources needed
8. Stakeholders
9. Risks
10. Internal and external communication
11. Purchasing
12. Requirements for change
13. Response to change.

How to Manage a Project in Support of a Strategic Plan

Developing a timeline is very important in managing a project in support of the strategic plan. Tools used in managing a project include a Gantt chart, the critical path method, critical path scheduling and the program evaluation and review technique (PERT).

Nurse executives should learn how to implement a strategic plan, particularly following the most important steps of:

1. Identifying goals
2. Creating a guide
3. Engaging staff
4. Making sure the budget and the strategic plan are in alignment
5. Conducting a pilot study or a number of them
6. Rolling out the plan with the help of well-trained and prepared staff
7. Monitoring and measuring progress
8. Making any appropriate modifications to the plan.

Nurse executives should also be familiar with the principles to be followed in monitoring the plans of action. These principles include comparing the prevailing status with the baseline, ascertaining if there is progress, making monitoring part of all programs, ensuring monitoring and evaluations are done concurrently and ensuring decisions are made on the basis of the information obtained from the monitoring. Another principle involves the monitoring methodology, which stipulates that a plan should be outlined in a clear manner and be consistently adhered to.

Any monitoring should observe confidentiality, focus on every primary stakeholder and be scheduled in a routine format. For proper monitoring, a matrix must be established, and resources should be distinguished from those allocated for other programs.

Nurse executives are expected to be conversant with the various approaches used to evaluate how well a program is progressing. These approaches include process assessment, assessment of outcomes, evaluation of the program impact and assessments of cost versus benefit or cost versus effectiveness.

Chapter 12: Summary of the Nurse Executive Position

This chapter is a brief review of all the information discussed in the preceding pages.

Nurse executives are nurses at the most senior level within health-care organizations. The 2017 publication of the *American Hospital Association Guide to the Health-Care Field* indicates that between 2013 and 2017, the number of qualified nurse executives almost doubled.

Responsibilities of Nurse Executives

Nurse executives mainly deal with the administrative aspects of health care in an organization. Their overall duty is to ensure that quality standards of service delivery are maintained in health-care institutions. However, their daily duties may vary depending on the type or size of a facility.

Financial accountability in health-care organizations falls under the jurisdiction of nurse executives as they are in charge of matters that involve managing and creating budgets. Nurse executives are also responsible for shaping health-care policies, designing and managing patient care, identifying loopholes in care services and developing new and more effective procedures.

Hiring, training and empowering staff for better service delivery is also part of nurse executives' mandate. They manage human resources and resolve conflicts that may arise within an organization. Nurse executives are expected to effectively communicate with different teams within the organization and to team up with them for the sake of developing partnerships and networks, which will be beneficial to the organization.

Nurse executives are responsible for delivering continuing education classes for their staff and improving the overall health of their patients, communities and families, while at the same time upholding ethical and professional principles.

The ability of nurse executives to collaborate with other health professionals, advocate for nursing staff and patients and develop quality health-care and wellness networks makes them key players in the smooth running of a health-care organization.

Personality Traits and Skills of Effective Nurse Executives

According to the American Organization of Nurse Executives, a successful nurse executive must have five main skills.

Communication & Relationship-Building Skills

Nurse executives must have the ability to communicate effectively and clearly with their team members, a trait that helps them resolve conflicts, hold productive discussions and provide a safe and trustworthy environment for staff.

They are also expected to produce oral and written presentations, represent the organization at councils and committees and continue building relationships with other professionals in and out of their institution.

Environmental Knowledge

Nurse executives are required to be highly knowledgeable not only in matters concerning clinical practices but also health-care economics, policies and governance, as well as research and data analysis. They are expected to understand evidence-based practice concepts and to make decisions based on various research findings in order to provide the most effective health-care services to patients.

It is also incumbent upon nurse executives to ensure their institutions are in compliance with specific laws and policies, like federal and state regulatory standards, the State Nurse Practice Act and the State Board of Nursing Regulations. There are instances where nurse executives are required to represent the nursing profession at board meetings.

Professionalism

It is important that nurse executives demonstrate utmost professionalism as they perform their duties. They are expected to abide by corporate policies, maintain their ethics, set work standards for their colleagues and coach others in developing their own career plans.

Leadership Skills

Nurse executives are expected to facilitate collaboration among different medical staff, promote a common vision for all within the organization, conduct community outreach, mentor potential nurse leaders and be effective in succession planning. All these activities require them to be assertive and to provide sound leadership to staff members and senior managers within an organization.

Business Skills

Nurse executives are not only required to understand the health-care demands from a management perspective, but also from the business perspective. They are responsible for managing financial resources; hiring, training and managing staff and conducting SWOT analyses. They must be adept at adapting to technological changes.

Experience and Education Requirements

To qualify for a nurse executive post, one needs to have a bachelor of science in nursing and must also have completed math and science prerequisites and have scored a 3.0 GPA. Among the courses in the nursing degree curriculum are pathophysiology, pharmacology, health assessment and foundations of professional nursing.

One needs to be a licensed RN before taking the National Council Licensure Examination to become a nurse executive.

With a bachelor's degree and sufficient practice as an RN, an individual should then obtain a master's degree. There is room to specialize in health-care administration, business administration or nursing in general. Completing these courses usually takes two to four years.

Nurse Executive Certifications

Nurse executives need to be certified by the ANCC in addition to being certified in Executive Nursing Practice through the AONE.

Continuing Education Courses

Nurse executives are expected to participate in continuing learning in order to maintain their credentials and to remain updated on changing nursing technology, research and practices.

Career Opportunities for Nurse Executives

The function of nurse executives has evolved from that of just providing nursing services in a health-care organization to providing all-round patient care. This change has led to an increase in career opportunities. In fact, many nursing schools and health-care organizations are now looking for nurse executives to occupy management positions within their organizations.

Other health care–affiliated industries, including insurance providers, are creating nurse executive posts that previously only existed in hospitals, home-based health agencies, health-care clinics and rehabilitation centers.

Nurse Executive Salaries

Because of the wide range of responsibilities that nurse executives are tasked with, they are normally well compensated. However, the salaries that individual executives earn depend on several factors, which include job location. As of 2017, the Bureau of Labor Statistics indicated the average yearly salary for health-care managers like nurse executives was $98,350.

Applying for Certification

The online certification test is available throughout the year. Once the test has been submitted, a candidate's results are sent back with indication of either a pass or a fail. If you do not pass on the first try, you are allowed to apply for a retest five days after the first testing date.

If you fail again, you can retest after sixty days. However, you can only retest three times in one year, and each of those times, you must meet ANCC eligibility requirements.

Certification Renewal

Nurse executives are required to renew their ANCC certification every five years, in order to demonstrate that they have expanded their professional knowledge, taken continual education courses and continually gained competence.

Test 1: Questions

(1) Generally, the clinics led by nurse executives are part of:

(A) Care organizations that are accountable

(B) Patient-centered medical homes

(C) Outpatient services

(D) Inpatient services

(2) When taking a census of inpatients over 24 hours, the count starts at:

(A) Noon

(B) 12:01 p.m.

(C) 12:01 a.m.

(D) Exactly midnight

(3) Which of the following services is covered under Medicare for those eligible, and is sometimes provided by home-based care health agencies?

(A) Services involving speech language pathology

(B) Homemaker services

(C) 24/7 home-based care

(D) Meal preparation or delivery

(4) For proper measure of throughput, it is best to begin with:

(A) Deciding on the measure to use

(B) Identifying benchmarks

(C) Determining target results

(D) Establishing a timeline

(5) What is the most suitable approach when, as a nurse executive, you have instituted unit-based self-scheduling for the purpose of sharing governance?

(A) Having the manager for every unit prepare the schedule

(B) Having individual staff members make personal schedules

(C) Having staff members negotiate among themselves and prepare the schedule together

(D) Having every unit form a committee that will prepare the schedule

(6) A newspaper reporter made an appointment with Jane, the nurse executive at St. Mary's Health Center, to discuss the center's initiatives toward enhancement of quality standards. What is the first thing Jane should do in preparation for the interview?

(A) Have notes ready for reference

(B) Prepare an official statement

(C) Have a discussion about it with the institution's person in charge of public relations

(D) Have a discussion about it with the health-care center's board of directors

(7) Judy, a nurse executive, is thinking of leaving primary nursing and taking up patient-based health care, where she will be able to work with a multidisciplinary team. What is the main shortcoming of patient-centered health care?

(A) The number of nursing staff required is higher.

(B) It is more expensive to implement.

(C) It is inconvenient to staff.

(D) It is inconvenient to patients.

(8) A nurse executive decides to prepare a pro forma operating budget prior to renovating a hospital. What does such a budget to accomplish?

(A) Estimate what the cost of the renovations is likely to be

(B) Monitor the expenses as they are incurred

(C) Obtain operating capital for use

(D) Distinguish costs of implementation from all other budget items

(9) There are plans to improve some processes at a health facility. Which of the following options is most expensive and most time consuming as a method of collecting data?

(A) Conducting surveys

(B) Conducting interviews

(C) Making observations

(D) Using a focus group

(10) An acute-care hospital plans to employ a pilot conversation program to replace the practice of documenting on paper and then processing via EHR. Such a program is best suited:

(A) For an independent unit that interacts minimally with different units

(B) For several units within the hospital

(C) For units that interact extensively with others

(D) For a unit whose size is as small as possible with regard to patient census

(11) For two-way communication to be effective, there needs to be:

(A) Timeliness

(B) Horizontal flow

(C) Feedback

(D) Vertical flow

(12) The beginning section of a business plan should comprise:

(A) Market-based strategies

(B) Products or services

(C) Market-related surveys

(D) Executive summaries

(13) What approach has the most effect when making significant changes in matters of policy and procedure?

(A) Being critical of previous approaches

(B) Appreciating the good in past approaches

(C) Ignoring previous approaches

(D) Emphasizing the benefits of the new plans

(14) Identify the initial stage in an organizational change as per Duck's Change Curve model of 2002.

(A) Preparation

(B) Fruition

(C) Stagnation

(D) Determination

(15) When trying to improve a process, it is appropriate to engage a blitz team for:

(A) Complicated projects that involve several departments

(B) Making quick fixes to problems that are localized

(C) Several projects

(D) Projects that are inexpensive

(16) Experienced nurses often note that those who are relatively young dislike working overtime and tend to take leaves of absence too often. This observation can be explained:

(A) As the young nurses lacking in motivation

(B) As the more experienced nurses being unfair to the younger ones

(C) As a mark of generational difference in the two groups' order of priorities

(D) As the younger nurses disliking the more experienced ones

(17) As far as innovation and other changes are concerned, the most important role of a nurse executive is:

(A) To develop concepts

(B) To carry out research on innovations

(C) To offer rewards for innovation

(D) To offer a vision

(18) When it is time to develop guidelines and pathways for clinical practice, the primary focus should be:

(A) The preferences of staff members

(B) Research pertaining to best health-care practices

(C) Internal research that is unit based

(D) Specialists' advice, like doctors

(19) Medicare's Hospital Compare website has information pertaining to:

(A) Consumerism

(B) Transparency

(C) Management

(D) Leadership

(20) When bedside reporting is initiated for the purposes of improving shift reporting, there is a likelihood that a problem could arise from nurses forgetting:

(A) To give thorough reports

(B) To keep their reports organized

(C) To ensure patients are addressed directly

(D) To give a report on every patient

(21) If regular surveys keep showing that patients are dissatisfied with the way nurses communicate with them, the problem can be best resolved by:

(A) Disseminating data widely

(B) Setting up competitions between nurses

(C) Penalizing nurses

(D) Training the nurses on how to communicate effectively

(22) The relationship-based care model focus on three major relationships—the nurse or any other health-care provider and the patient and family, the individual and another party. Who is that other party?

(A) The public in general

(B) The health provider's colleagues

(C) The institution's administration

(D) The physicians

(23) It is the opinion of a certain nurse executive that newly recruited RNs should undergo an intensive orientation program. The first thing the nurse executive should do to upgrade the existing orientation program is to:

(A) Take a survey of the existing members of the nursing staff

(B) Put forward a proposal to make changes

(C) Hold a meeting with supervisors of all units to get their input

(D) Collect information regarding other orientation programs

(24) When there is a service recovery program in place that seeks to increase patients' satisfaction with the care they receive, the initial response whenever a patient encounters a problem should be:

(A) To accept there is a problem and offer an apology for it

(B) To solve the problem quietly, without alerting the patient

(C) To offer some form of compensation for the patient

(D) To identify the person who caused the problem

(25) Sharing governance can be done through partnership councils, a form of governance known for:

(A) Having its sole focus on nursing

(B) Having nurses share decision-making with physicians

(C) Involving patients and their families

(D) Involving staff from every level and area of an organization

(26) In persuasive communication, the element considered to be of utmost importance is:

(A) Use of suitable body language

(B) Having a good understanding of your audience

(C) Having benefits well outlined

(D) Ensuring credibility is established

(27) Often the manner of communication with surgery patients prior to and after the operation has been found to be inconsistent, so as a nurse executive, your suggestion is for staff to rely on scripting. When scripting, once introductions have been made, the words spoken soon after should address:

(A) General niceties in conversation

(B) Any questions a patient may have

(C) The topic and purpose

(D) How comfortable the patient feels

(28) If disaster strikes, what should be the first strategy instituted to ensure a hospital's surge capacity is increased?

(A) Identifying patients who can be safely discharged early

(B) Placing of additional beds in rooms normally allocated for private use

(C) Recommending not accepting patients in the emergency room unless they are clients associated with the disaster

(D) Transferring patients to open rooms

(29) If you want to mainly target the demographic of patients in their twenties, the most effective means of communication is:

(A) Text messages

(B) Email

(C) Postal mail

(D) Landline telephones

(30) There are several nurses working at an institution who had been away for some years to tend to their young children. This style of career used by the nurses can be termed:

(A) Linear

(B) Steady state

(C) Spiral

(D) Entrepreneurial or transient

(31) As per tort law, any nurse who prevents a mentally sound patient from leaving a hospital on his/her own even when the patient does not pose a risk to anyone, including himself/herself, is liable for:

(A) Committing battery

(B) Committing assault

(C) Kidnapping

(D) Engaging in false imprisonment

(32) Which method can a nurse executive with half of the staff close to retirement follow in a bid to convince members to postpone retirement and increase retention?

(A) Offer monetary bonuses

(B) Offer flexible schedules and assignments

(C) Offer to pair the nurses with staff members who are younger

(D) Request that they postpone their retirement

(33) Identify the best option from those listed below if the nurse executive' intention is to increase input and gain support from members of the community.

(A) Using focus groups

(B) Carrying out patient-based surveys

(C) Forming patient/family advisory councils

(D) Interviewing patients

(34) Which of the following is an alternative used to refer to total factor productivity?

(A) Entropic productivity

(B) Human resource productivity

(C) Statistical stability productivity

(D) Multifactor productivity

(35) Which of the following is true regarding productivity?

(A) Many different factors can have a positive or negative impact on productivity.

(B) JCAHO has mathematical methods and standards that it uses to measure productivity.

(C) The decrease in cost of equipment and supplies causes a decrease in productivity.

(D) The mix and size of a workforce is the main factor that usually affects productivity.

(36) During orientations, what type of content gives adults the most motivation to learn?

(A) Content addressing their future learning requirements

(B) Information addressing their future career goals

(C) Content addressing their short-term learning needs

(D) Information addressing their immediate career goals

(37) Which of the following statements is true about the Patient Protection and Affordable Care Act?

(A) In 2011, the act was repealed.

(B) The act was implemented fully in 2011.

(C) The act became law in 2010.

(D) In 2011, the act was declared unconstitutional.

(38) A health corporation's total assets are valued at a billion dollars, and its total liabilities are valued at $754,739,089. Using this data, calculate the corporation's asset/liability ratio.

(A) 0.75

(B) 1.32

(C) 0.76

(D) 1.33

(39) Which of the following statements regarding orientation is correct?

(A) Orientation should last for two days.

(B) Orientation is usually a process, not an event.

(C) Orientation should only be conducted in a physical classroom setting.

(D) Orientation should start a week after hiring.

(40) James notices a negative variance in operating expenses when carrying out a monthly departmental budget review. After analyzing this variance, he determines that it was caused by overtime pay. Which action should James take?

(A) He should inform his immediate supervisor of the salary savings.

(B) He should ignore the variance, since it may not even be accurate.

(C) He should congratulate the staff for keeping the overtime salaries to a minimum.

(D) He should work with the staff to identify ways to reduce the need to work overtime.

(41) Which of the following lists the correct stages of the recruitment process?

(A) Job analysis, screening, sourcing, and selection

(B) Assessment, implementation, planning, and evaluation

(C) Job analysis, implementation, planning, and evaluation

(D) Assessment, screening, sourcing, and selection

(42) Almost every health-care institution uses a computerized accounting system. Identify the system's major benefit.

(A) It reduces staff and salaries.

(B) It proves that a nonprofit facility is not making any profit.

(C) It complies with the United States Paperwork Reduction Act.

(D) It ensures that data collected is accurate and helps nurse executives make informed decisions.

(43) Which of these hospital documents has information that is helpful in carrying out successful interviews?

(A) The Human Resources Employee Manual

(B) The departmental budget

(C) The philosophy, goals, and mission of the health facility

(D) Clerical and ancillary employee job description

(44) Which of the following statements is true about the Indian Health Service?

(A) It was founded in 1965 under the United States Bureau of Indian Affairs.

(B) It was founded in 1955 under the United States Bureau of Indian Affairs.

(C) It was founded in 1955 under the United States Department of Health and Human Services.

(D) It was founded in 1965 under the United States Department of Health and Human Services.

(45) Which of the following candidates best qualifies for a job in a hospital?

(A) A candidate who is unqualified but demonstrates a great willingness to learn the job

(B) A member of a minority Christian faith group who practices his or her faith

(C) An overqualified individual whose qualifications far exceed the job expectations

(D) A disabled person who is minimally qualified and is covered under the Americans with Disabilities Act

(46) Which of the following interview questions can be said to be open ended?

(A) Have you read the philosophy of our hospital?

(B) Are you ready to work long hours over the weekends?

(C) Was it difficult to locate our hospital?

(D) Tell us a bit about your accomplishments and aspirations.

(47) Which performance improvement point may be investigated during a quality-and-performance improvement activity?

(A) Process: The patient's compliance

(B) Structure: The patient's satisfaction

(C) Structure: The number of patients with MRSA infections

(D) Outcome: Severity of any falls

(48) During orientation, which piece of equipment must every organization teach its new employees how to properly use?

(A) Fire extinguishers

(B) The vending machine in the cafeteria

(C) The bedside computer system

(D) An emergency shutoff valve

(49) Which of the following shows the correct steps involved in a budgeting process?

(A) Defining the problem, determining and implementing an option, and evaluating

(B) Assessing, planning, evaluating, and implementing

(C) Variance analysis, determining and implementing an option, and evaluating

(D) Gathering data, planning, coming up with a budget, negotiating or revising, and evaluating

(50) Which of the following correctly identifies the qualities of a successful orientation process?

(A) It is timely, complete, effective, and appropriate.

(B) It is brief, timely, complete, and costly.

(C) It is conducted while providing care to a patient.

(D) It is complete and rated favorably by the learners.

(51) Which is the main characteristic of an operating budget that distinguishes it from a capital budget?

(A) It addresses only fixed and variable costs.

(B) It addresses only staff salaries, compensation, and benefits.

(C) It addresses the unit renovation cost to meet JCAHO standards.

(D) Operating budgets are used for patient care equipment with costs less than $1,000.

(52) What type of reimbursement is set by the diagnosis-related groups?

(A) Medicaid retrospective compensation

(B) Medicare prospective compensation

(C) Medicare retrospective compensation

(D) Medicaid prospective compensation

(53) Identify the situation with the potential to cause conflict in an organization.

(A) Unclear roles within empowered organizations

(B) A staff member who is not able to prioritize tasks

(C) A staff member who is not able to resolve an ethical dilemma

(D) Staff members who are not able to resolve scheduling and staffing conflicts

(54) James is leading a process that involves the introduction of new technology meant to improve the way medical information in a facility is handled. Which of these staff behaviors can help him determine whether staff members are resisting change?

(A) Reemergence

(B) Communicability

(C) Indifference

(D) Equilibrium

(55) Which is the most ideal intervention to utilize when two parties in conflict turn their frustration into anger?

(A) Hire a moderator who can hold group sessions with the parties in a bid to resolve the conflict

(B) Clarify the differences according to the individuals' goals and priorities

(C) Apply the law-and-order approach that includes the use of procedures and policies as the basis of conflict resolution

(D) Take an autocratic decision-making approach in order to protect the affected staff's well-being

(56) Which of these mentorship techniques used in professional development programs involves the mentor sending a mentee into a complex situation that the mentee has not experienced before?

(A) Sowing

(B) Synthesizing

(C) Analyzing

(D) Catalyzing

(57) Which of the following leads to poor problem-solving?

(A) Failure to define an issue or problem accurately

(B) An attitude of inaction

(C) Failure to have alternative causes of action

(D) Change resistance from a group

(58) Which of these tools effectively analyzes the steps taken when processes are complex?

(A) Flowchart

(B) Pareto chart

(C) Histogram

(D) Fishbone diagram

(59) What is the benefit of reverse mentoring for an organization and individuals with regard to professional development?

(A) Managers who are less experienced get a chance to learn through the senior managers.

(B) It offers the chance to relearn certain skills from younger mentors.

(C) Mentees receive new and advanced techniques and perspectives.

(D) There are no benefits from this type of mentoring.

(60) Which of these circumstances shows there is likely to be no resolution to a conflict?

(A) The conflict is caused by the need to distribute scarce resources.

(B) Staff feel that their organization does not grant them autonomy.

(C) Staff feel that their organization does not care about their lack of satisfaction.

(D) Conflict frequently reoccurs.

(61) The terms and processes associated with enhancement of performance and quality have continued to evolve over the years. Which of the following represents a process that correctly matches its previous and currently used term, respectively?

(A) Performance improvement, quality improvement

(B) Quality improvement, quality control

(C) Continuous quality assurance, quality assurance

(D) Total quality management, quality management

(62) Which of the following patients is most prone to medical error?

(A) A diabetic lady who is not compliant but is alert

(B) A man with a language barrier

(C) An adolescent who has just survived a car crash

(D) An elderly woman using a walker

(63) A root-cause analysis has to be credible and thorough. What needs to be done for the analysis to be deemed credible?

(A) All the risk points must be identified.

(B) There must be a set of questions that are meant to investigate the "why."

(C) The causes that are "not applicable" must also be explained.

(D) The analysis should last for at least six hours.

(64) Which of the following represents the performance improvement structure of a magnet hospital?

(A) A professional autonomy

(B) A flattened and decentralized organizational structure

(C) A hierarchal organizational structure

(D) An independent decision-making structure

(65) Empowerment of the nursing staff sometimes causes fear among nursing managers and supervisors. How can such fear be best described?

(A) Fear of losing delegation

(B) Fear of lower productivity

(C) Fear of losing control

(D) Fear of compromised health-care quality

(66) Which of the following is the main focus of every relationship within a health-care setup?

(A) Upper management

(B) Consumers

(C) The agency

(D) Middle management

(67) Which of the following is a goal for a long-term care institution, addressed in the 2012 National Patient Safety Goal program?

(A) Anticoagulants and their effectiveness

(B) Intravenous therapy safety

(C) Preventing wrong-site surgeries

(D) Using two unique resident identifiers

(68) Which of the following statements regarding clinical information systems' technology programs is true?

(A) The programs are being introduced in health care.

(B) They have very limited uses.

(C) They are created by many companies.

(D) They are not useful in strategic management.

(69) When extinguishing electrical fires, which kind of fire extinguisher should you use?

(A) Class B

(B) Class C

(C) Class D

(D) Class A

(70) Which term best describes the process that seeks to eliminate the gap existing between the present situation and the situation as it ought to be?

(A) Decision-making

(B) Problem-solving

(C) Empowerment

(D) Divergent thinking

(71) Which of the following decision-making models consumes a lot of time but results in the best decisions?

(A) Optimizing

(B) Normative

(C) Descriptive

(D) Satisficing

(72) HIPAA requires health-care facilities to carry out risk analyses using patient information technology as a strategic management measure. How often should such analyses be done?

(A) Every day

(B) Every week

(C) Every year

(D) Continuously

(73) Identify the change theory that involves developing relationships, diagnosing a problem, and subsequently acquiring the required resources.

(A) Lippitt's, Watson's, and Westley's theory

(B) Lewin's Force Field Analysis theory

(C) Roger's Six Phases of Planned Change

(D) Havelock's Six Phases of Planned Change

(74) Identify the five different modes of conflict resolution.

(A) Avoiding, accommodating, consulting, collaborating, and commanding

(B) Collaborating, competing, compromising, affinitizing, and avoiding

(C) Collaborating, compromising, avoiding, competing, and accommodating

(D) Avoiding, collaborating, accommodating, collegiality, and consulting

(75) Which of the following information should be presented using PowerPoint slides?

(A) A narrative

(B) Learning objectives

(C) Narrative accounts

(D) A policy

(76) What course of action should you take if a tornado watch alert is issued in your region?

(A) Evacuate the patients outdoors to prevent them from getting injured by broken glass

(B) Move the patients to the building's highest floor

(C) There is nothing you can do since the tornado has already formed

(D) Move all the patients away from the windows and wait for further instructions

(77) Which certification from the American Nurses Credentialing Center determines whether a nurse in the information technology field is competent?

(A) Nursing Informatics

(B) Nursing Technology

(C) Health Technology

(D) Health Information

(78) Which law requires employers to identify and use safe medical devices in order to ensure staff safety at a health-care facility?

(A) The Bloodborne Pathogens Act

(B) The Needlestick Safety and Prevention Act

(C) The Occupational Safety and Health Administration Act (OSHA)

(D) The Occupational Safety Act

(79) Which of these practices can help you effectively prevent procrastination, especially when you are dealing with a large or complex project?

(A) Select the easiest task and do it first

(B) Understand that your procrastination is a result of overworking

(C) Select the interesting tasks and do them first

(D) Determine the factors that are causing the procrastination

(80) Which of the following identifies the steps involved in a project management process in their correct order?

(A) Storming, forming, norming

(B) Forming, storming, norming

(C) Initiation, planning, implementation, monitoring, completion

(D) Planning, initiation, implementation, monitoring, completion

(81) Which of the following choices represents the different engineering controls used to promote workplace safety?

(A) Solidifying of blood

(B) Disposing of needles or other sharp objects properly

(C) Adhering to set standard precautions

(D) Using personal protective equipment properly

(82) Which United States military response team plan should be included in a health-care facility's contingency plan?

(A) Workplace violence contingency plan

(B) Bioterrorism contingency plan

(C) Storm contingency plan

(D) Flood contingency plan

(83) What is the main purpose of having contingency plans within a business?

(A) They enhance efficiency, timeliness, and effectiveness of services despite external environmental changes.

(B) They enhance efficiency, timeliness, and effectiveness of services despite internal environment changes.

(C) They help in maintaining quality and reducing redundancies despite constant changes in the internal environment.

(D) They help in maintaining quality and reducing risk despite constant changes in the external and internal environment.

(84) Which of the following actions applies when using fogging as the communication technique of choice in managing criticism?

(A) Using distraction as a way to avoid acknowledging criticism

(B) Encouraging other people to communicate in an assertive manner

(C) Using intimidation as a way of redirecting the conversation

(D) Agreeing in principle and receiving criticism without turning defensive

(85) Which decision-making model is a nurse executive likely to utilize when implementing a nursing program that must be evaluated after its implementation?

(A) Collegial model

(B) Bureaucratic model

(C) Garbage-can model

(D) Cybernetic model

(86) Which of the following questions is not acceptable to ask a prospective employee during an interview?

(A) Do you believe you can handle the duties that come with this position?

(B) Do you have authorization to work here in the United States?

(C) Do you have children? If so, how many?

(D) Have you previously worked for our hospital under another name?

(87) A patient visited the hospital every week with different complaints, and these views were reflected in the patient's records. The nursing staff classified the man as a service abuser and an attention seeker. One day the patient came in complaining of abdominal pains and received minimal treatment. Soon he was discharged. A while later, the staff was informed that the man had an internal blockage that required surgery, and it was performed at another facility. With pending litigation, the defense attorney reviewed the existing nursing documentation to understand the case against the nurses. What were the nurses likely charged with based on the given events?

(A) Harassment

(B) Slander

(C) Unintentional tort

(D) Libel

(88) For which service are minors in 50 US states allowed to give informed consent?

(A) Abortion

(B) Contraceptive services

(C) HIV testing and HIV treatment

(D) STD testing and STD treatment, excluding HIV

(89) Why are paternalistic actions not compatible with nursing ethics?

(A) They decrease the nurse's authority.

(B) They reduce the nurse's accountability.

(C) They diminish the patient's autonomy.

(D) They reduce the ethical obligation.

(90) Which delivery model used in nursing care gives a nurse an all-day-responsibility over a patient's rights, beginning when the patient is admitted and ending when he/she is discharged?

(A) Modular nursing

(B) Team nursing

(C) Primary nursing

(D) Functional nursing

(91) What does the patient classification system measure?

(A) Acuity level

(B) How satisfied customers are

(C) How safe patients are

(D) Variations in performance

(92) What was the initial purpose of developing diagnosis-related groups?

(A) To provide funds for private insurance firms

(B) To determine the benefits of prescription drugs

(C) To facilitate sliding-scale reimbursements for Medicare beneficiaries

(D) To determine Medicare reimbursements at a set fee

(93) At which level are programs that deal with disposal of medical waste regulated?

(A) State level

(B) Federal level

(C) Community level

(D) Local level

(94) According to the Patient Self-Determination Act, what are federally funded hospitals required to do?

(A) Treat patients who have no insurance

(B) Provide appropriate accommodation for patients who have disabilities

(C) Protect patients by maintaining regulations that make nurses accountable

(D) Provide patients with a notice in written form, concerning the right they have to make decisions pertaining to their treatment

(95) Which business analysis technique are nurse executives likely to use in strategic planning?

(A) SWOT analysis

(B) VPEC-T analysis

(C) PC analysis

(D) Moscow analysis

(96) Which budget-making method requires that there be an exhaustive review, as well as justification for expenditures, before any resources can be allocated?

(A) Zero-based budgeting (ZBB)

(B) Activity-based budgeting (ABB)

(C) Priority-based budgeting (PBB)

(D) Incremental budgeting

(97) From which budget are funds allocated if they are intended for the replacement of broken beds in a health-care unit?

(A) The marketing budget

(B) The capital budget

(C) The operational budget

(D) The labor budget

(98) In an effort to establish higher standards, what process involves comparing the services provided in a hospital to the most efficient practices in other industries providing similar services?

(A) Market research

(B) Networking

(C) Benchmarking

(D) Quantitative research

(99) Which aspect of a nursing process can be delegated under supervision?

(A) Intervention

(B) Evaluation

(C) Planning

(D) Assessment

(100) Which requirement, according to Occupational Safety and Health Administration laws, should any new employee providing direct care to patients comply with?

(A) Undergo a TB test every year

(B) Receive the three-shot hepatitis B vaccine

(C) Get a titer after the hepatitis B vaccination

(D) Be evaluated by a health-care giver in case of a needlestick injury

(101) Who worked alongside Clara Barton as she took care of black soldiers who were wounded in the Civil War, and also helped slaves escape through the Underground Railroad?

(A) Harriet Tubman

(B) Albert Einstein

(C) Florence Harding

(D) Peter Cooper

(102)Which of the following nurses was born into a slave family and is remembered for improving sanitation for black soldiers and providing them with food and clothing?

(A) George Thompson

(B) Dr. Joseph DeeLee

(C) Sojourner Truth

(D) Mary Breckinridge

(103)Which of the following people reduced the workday for student nurses from 10 to eight hours?

(A) Isabel Hampton Robb

(B) Mary Adelaide

(C) Linda Richards

(D) Mildred Montag

(104)Which of the following people designed the FNS and the first school for training midwives?

(A) Mary Breckinridge

(B) Lavinia Dock

(C) Florence Nightingale

(D) Archimedes

(105) Which of the following people carried out a study that led to the introduction of the associate degree in nurse education?

(A) Mary Seacole

(B) Margaret Sanger

(C) Elizabeth G. Neill

(D) Mildred Montag

(106)Which of the following individuals was a nurse leader who contributed to the enhancement of community nursing even as she fought for women's rights?

(A) Adelaide Nutting

(B) Lavinia Dock

(C) Mary E. Mahoney

(D) Lillian Wald

(107) Which of the following people developed a theory that a patient is someone who needs help in regaining independence?

(A) Susie K. Taylor

(B) Virginia Henderson

(C) Mary E. Walker

(D) Dr. Hildegard

(108) Which of the following was a pioneering African American nurse in America?

(A) Mary Mahoney

(B) Mabel K. Staupers

(C) Louyse Bourgeois

(D) Florence Nightingale

(109) Which psychiatric nurse developed the theory that describes the nurse-client relationship?

(A) Rebecca L. Crumpler

(B) Elizabeth Blackwell

(C) Isabella Baumfree

(D) Hildegard Peplau

(110) Who was the first person to qualify as a trained nurse in America and also contributed immensely in developing nurse education by taking her campaigns from one hospital to another?

(A) Sara J. Baker

(B) Hazel W. Johnson

(C) Melinda Ann (Linda) Richards

(D) H. E. Peplau

(111) Who started the first clinic for birth control in the United States?

(A) Mary E. Pennington

(B) Margaret Sanger

(C) Lady Bird Johnson

(D) Sojourner Truth

(112) Who established a nurse service for neighborhoods in New York City as an example of public health nursing?

(A) Lillian Wald

(B) Dolly Parton

(C) Florence Seibert

(D) Christiane Reimann

(113) What happened in 1832 that highlighted the nobility of the nursing profession?

(A) A cholera outbreak occurred in Ireland, where nurses from the Sisters of Mercy were selfless in helping patients.

(B) President Andrew Jackson praised nurses during a big conference.

(C) Samuel Morse revealed that the motivation behind the development of the Morse Code was the work nurses were doing in remote areas of the country.

(D) Nothing significant occurred.

(114) In the 1840s and 1850s, the Sisters of Charity became known for their charitable actions. What were some of their most prominent activities?

(A) Feeding youth and working toward reducing teenage pregnancy

(B) Fetching water and cooking for WWII soldiers

(C) Visiting the sick at home and later starting a hospital in Cincinnati

(D) Opening a surgical unit in Detroit and giving out free medicines

(115) The first formally trained US nurse was a student of the Florence Nightingale Training School, but she graduated from the New England Hospital for Women & Children. Where was this hospital located?

(A) New Orleans

(B) Washington, D.C.

(C) Boston

(D) Chicago

(116) Male nurses began rendering care during the 1090 crusades. What were these nurses part of?

(A) Military nursing orders

(B) Navy lifesavers

(C) Protestant youth groups

(D) None of the above

(117) Which war did Florence Nightingale's nursing efforts impact the most?

(A) World War I

(B) World War II

(C) The Vietnam War

(D) The Crimean War

(118) Which law was passed in 2002 to address the shortage of nurses through recruitment initiatives and retention?

(A) The Americas Partnership for Nursing Education Act

(B) The Model Nursing Practice Act

(C) The Nurse Reinvestment Act

(D) The National Nurse Act

(119) Which statement about privacy rules in the Health Insurance Portability and Accountability Act is true?

(A) During a public health emergency, covered entities may disclose protected medical information without the authorization of an individual.

(B) When medical information is transcribed, covered entities are allowed to retain that information in its tape-recorded version.

(C) Covered entities are authorized to impose a fee for the search and retrieval of copies of any medical records upon request.

(D) Individuals are restricted from accessing their medical records following clinical trials.

(120) Which of the following choices is a quantitative research method that looks at statistical analysis from different research studies on a given topic for the purposes of investigating the study features and then integrating the findings?

(A) Survey

(B) Metanalysis

(C) Methodological study

(D) Assessment of needs

(121) Which of the following is a characteristic of federal regulation regarding an institutional review board?

(A) When voting on a complex issue, a specialist may be invited.

(B) The board members may all be from one profession.

(C) The board must have a member who has no affiliation with the institution.

(D) Any member whose main concerns are not scientific should not be included.

(122) According to health-care institutions, customers are either internal or external. Which of the following can be considered external customers?

(A) Hospital administrators

(B) Hospital-based physicians

(C) Managed-care companies on contract

(D) Patient care providers

(123) A nursing staff was recently informed that their surgical unit would be moved to a different building within the campus so that construction of another surgical unit could begin. Some of the staff verbally complained that the smaller unit they were to move to would accommodate less staff, which in turn would compromise patient care. As a reliable change agent, what should you do?

(A) Avoid acknowledging the complaints and go ahead with the move to discourage any further negative feedback

(B) Call for a meeting with the department and notify the staff that this is a mandatory move and is not debatable

(C) Involve the staff in the transition and hold a staff meeting to provide further information, even as you welcome any feedback

(D) Ask the staff to write a formal complaint, which is to be forwarded to the administration

(124) Which conflict resolution style involves an active attempt by both parties to find a solution that can satisfy the goals of the two parties?

(A) Compromise

(B) Avoidance

(C) Collaboration

(D) Accommodation

(125) Which of the following statements deals with exempt employees under the Fair Labor Standards Act?

(A) Employees working for more than 40 hours in a week must receive overtime payment.

(B) Employees must get at least one break after every four hours of work.

(C) Employees should not be subjected to a minimum wage, since they are salaried.

(D) Employees must be given seven holidays per year if they work 40 hours per week.

(126) Which of the following activities is not required of an accredited hospital according to the Joint Commission's Sentinel Event Policy?

(A) Conducting a root-cause analysis in 45 days upon learning of any reviewable sentinel events

(B) Reporting all specified sentinel events

(C) Developing a course of action and responding accordingly to a sentinel event

(D) Defining all the events in the facility to be reviewed in accordance with the Sentinel Event Policy

(127) According to the Joint Commission's Sentinel Event Policy, which of these events is a reviewable sentinel event?

(A) An employee's death caused by exposure to a blood-borne pathogen

(B) A patient's death due to early discharge that was contrary to medical advice

(C) Fall of a patient that led to permanent and total loss of limb function

(D) A suicide attempt that was not successful and did not cause major loss of bodily function

(128) According to the Joint Commission's National Patient Safety Goal, which of the following is a "do not use" symbol in medicine orders?

(A) 0.1 mg

(B) 1.0 mg

(C) 1 mL

(D) 1 mg

(129) Which of the following elements is not proof that a nurse should be held accountable for malpractice?

(A) The nurse breached care standards.

(B) There was an existing patient-nurse relationship.

(C) The actions of the nurse were directly connected to the injury the patient sustained.

(D) The patient suffered damage or an injury.

(130) Which option, according to HIPAA, does not allow for protected health data to be disclosed for clinical research?

(A) The de-identification of protected health data

(B) The subject signing informed consent

(C) The subject signing a valid privacy rule authorization

(D) A privacy board or institutional review board granting a waiver

(131) Which personal information does not require removal during the process of de-identifying?

(A) The state

(B) Birthdate

(C) Email addresses

(D) Social Security number

(132) According to the five-stage model known as Tuckman's stages, which is the stage during which the leader clarifies the roles and rules of working together and the team members start to commit to the goals of the team?

(A) Storming

(B) Norming

(C) Forming

(D) Performing

(133) Which leadership power is characterized by followers complying because it is their belief that the leader has authority to lead, and not because of rewards or fear of possible negative consequences?

(A) Expert power

(B) Referent power

(C) Coercive power

(D) Legitimate power

(134) Which behavior is manifested by a preceptor who gives orientees partial information or incomplete answers, and does so in a patronizing tone, contending that the information is not important to the orientees at that stage?

(A) Intimidation

(B) Clinical violence

(C) Lateral violence

(D) Verbal abuse

(135) Which infectious disease requires a medical practitioner to complete a Standard Centers for Disease Control case form?

(A) Listeriosis

(B) Histoplasmosis

(C) Leptospirosis

(D) Campylobacteriosis

(136) Which division in the Department of Health and Human Services investigates Medicare fraud?

(A) Office of Global Health Affairs

(B) Office of Medicare Hearings and Appeals

(C) Office of Intergovernmental Affairs

(D) Office of the Inspector General

(137) When designing a staffing plan, which factors are assessed as per the American Nurses Association Principles for Nurse Staffing?

(A) Available technology

(B) Staff skill level and experience

(C) The patient population

(D) Nursing hours for each patient day

(138) Which of the following choices represents centralized decision-making?

(A) Forming a committee that is made up of nurses to participate in a quality-improvement initiative

(B) Staff members participating in a self-scheduling activity

(C) Nurses using the Primary Nursing Model to provide care

(D) The nurse manager approving all new employees through the hospital's nurse executive

(139) A unit manager informed a nurse executive that she planned to resign because she could not meet the reduced stuff budgeting expectations. What cognitive distortion does this unit manager have?

(A) Catastrophizing

(B) Fortune-telling

(C) All-or-nothing thinking

(D) Disqualifying the positives

(140) Which of the following statements regarding the Belmont Report is accurate?

(A) It provides regulations that protect human subjects during research.

(B) It is founded on the principles of autonomy, justice, and respect.

(C) It identifies the principles of ethics that serve as the basis for establishing the Health and Human Services' regulations meant to protect human subjects.

(D) It makes recommendations for Health and Human Services administrative action on the mistreatment of human subjects during research.

(141) Which of the following activities may not be banned by the employment laws and regulations of the United States' Equal Employment Opportunity Commission?

(A) Recruiting orally, which may result in attracting a similar workforce

(B) Advertising employment opportunities that are exclusively for female staff

(C) Requesting applicants provide a photograph during the first stages of the hiring process

(D) Reducing older workers' benefits in order to match younger workers' cost of benefits

(142) What is the ultimate goal of Healthy People 2020?

(A) To track national disease data for a period of 10 years

(B) To compile evidence-based information on issues related to public health

(C) To prevent disease and promote health for every American

(D) To educate public health staff on the main causes of illnesses

(143) Which insurance covers an employer against litigation that results from a work-related accident caused by an employee's negligence?

(A) Public Liability Insurance

(B) Keyman Insurance

(C) Worker's Compensation Insurance

(D) Employer's Liability Insurance

(144) What part of the Medicare program provides for a private health insurance option?

(A) Part B

(B) Part A

(C) Part D

(D) Part C

(145) Which of the following conditions or procedures is no longer allowed by the Deficit Reduction Act?

(A) Blood administration

(B) Bypass surgery

(C) Air embolism

(D) Urinary tract infection

(146) Which of the following option does OSHA require be included in an Exposure Control Plan?

(A) Procedures for evaluating exposure events

(B) Data sheets pertaining to safety issues and a full list of dangerous chemicals

(C) Exposure determination and identifying job classifications

(D) Implementing exposure control methods

(147) Which quality improvement method is used in identifying and preventing potential problems?

(A) Barrier analysis

(B) Root-cause analysis

(C) Failure mode and effects analysis

(D) Causal factor analysis

(148) Which of the following analysis tools uses the 80/20 rule, which suggests that 80 percent of problems are usually caused by 20 percent of causes?

(A) Gantt chart

(B) Pareto chart

(C) Flowchart

(D) Run chart

(149) Which of the following statements describes how a Gantt chart differs from a PERT chart?

(A) A Gantt chart is more ideal for a large project than a PERT chart.

(B) A Gantt is a form of bar chart, while a PERT chart is a form of flowchart.

(C) In a Gantt chart, the arrows in between the activity nodes represent activity times.

(D) It is easier to follow dependencies between different activities in a Gantt chart than it is in a PERT chart.

(150) Which of the following nonprofit organizations accredits medical groups, physicians, and health plans and provides other programs, like multicultural health-care distinction and credential verification?

(A) Council of Accreditation

(B) Joint Commission

(C) National Committee for Quality Assurance

(D) National Nonprofit Accreditation Center

Test 1: Answers and Explanations

(1) (C) Outpatient services

Many of the clinics led by nurses offer outpatient services, and they mostly treat members of the community who have chronic ailments. Such clinics have hours of operation, which include evenings and weekends, in order to make services accessible to as many people as possible.

(2) (C) 12:01 a.m.

Every patient counted during the census is representative of one inpatient service day. The number of inpatient beds found to be available in a given period is termed bed-count days. (Inpatient service days ÷ inpatient bed-count days) x 100 produces the rate of inpatient bed occupancy.

(3) (A) Services involving speech language pathology

In order to qualify for home-based care, a patient must be certified homebound by a physician and be intermittently in need of skilled health care, such as physical or occupational therapy, from a nurse. Note that a patient can be homebound and still be able to attend a day-care program for adults.

(4) (B) Identifying benchmarks

The term “throughput” is used in reference to the total quantity of data, information, or products that can successfully be put through a system. At one point the term was applied solely in reference to processing of data, but now it is applied to products of other processes as well.

(5) (D) Having every unit form a committee that will prepare the schedule

The committee is expected to ensure that staffing is adequate, even as it tries to exhibit fairness and accommodate the desires of individual staff members. The committee should refrain from making seniority a priority during self-scheduling, as such a tendency can make other staff members resentful.

(6) (C) Have a discussion about it with the institution's person in charge of public relations

Consulting with PR personnel ensures that every member of the hospital says only complimentary things. The PR person may advise you, for example, to emphasize patient care rather than the savings the hospital makes by reducing costs.

(7) (B) It is more expensive to implement.

Among the increased costs are those incurred when moving services as close as possible to patients. For example, it may become necessary for individual units to have their own occupational therapist.

(8) (A) Estimate what the cost of the renovations is likely to be

Although the information in a pro forma operating budget may not be actual, when that information is of good quality, such a budget is helpful in revealing costs that would not otherwise stand out, thereby preventing unexpected costs that might take the hospital by surprise.

(9) (B) Conducting interviews

The reason conducting interviews is so expensive and time consuming is that these are done on a one-on-one basis, and it takes time to record them and quantify the information collected. There is also the cost of compensating the interviewers, and probably some cost is incurred beforehand to train them so that the process is consistent.

(10) (A) For an independent unit that interacts minimally with different units

Units whose interactions are extensive cannot properly use some of the features of EHR. It is crucial to note the importance of monitoring any pilot process that has been implemented. If successful, the program can be of great use in training other staff.

(11) (C) Feedback

Irrespective of whether the communication is between a leader and a subordinate (termed vertical) or between individual staff members (termed horizontal), feedback is necessary. One must always receive a response after relaying a message. So, a nurse executive should not only expect a request or an answer to a question he/she poses, he/she should also respond to received messages.

(12) (D) Executive summaries

That part should be concise and inclusive of a business proposal's major elements in the form of an outline. The target customers should also be included, along with the products or services offered and the business goals.

(13) (B) Appreciating the good in past approaches

The value you identify in approaches used in the past can be helpful in laying the foundation for the intended changes. Also, if you focus on criticizing approaches used in the past, you are likely to get resistance from those who preferred the previous way of doing things.

(14) (C) Stagnation

The order is stagnation, preparation, implementation, and determination. In stagnation, people are not interested in change. In the preparation stage, they become both anxious and hopeful, and it helps the change process if people can buy into the idea. In the third stage, people appreciate probable benefits to them, while the fourth stage brings disappointment if success is not met.

(15) (B) Making quick fixes to problems that are localized

Such a team normally comprises staff members directly involved in implementing the process, like those working in the unit where there is a process to be enhanced. The team may be an ad hoc one, formed solely to address the problem unique to that particular unit.

(16) (C) As a mark of generational differences in the two groups' order of priorities

The reason such complaints arise is that the older generation has, over the years, been willing to work longer hours at the expense of relaxation or recreational time, but the younger generation is eager to have a better work-life balance.

(17) (D) To offer a vision

Such vision encompasses articulating the necessity for innovation; appreciating and rewarding fresh ideas; providing resources required for change; treating failures as enlightening experiences; providing ways to communicate ideas; providing guidelines to encourage fresh, innovative ideas; encouraging research committees; and giving public credit to innovators.

(18) (B) Research pertaining to best health-care practices

Even if physicians and other specialists have great input, their view may be influenced by what is familiar to them. The same case applies to members of staff, who may state their preference on the basis of what they are familiar with rather than what is best.

(19) (B) Transparency

Medicare's Hospital Compare website provides information pertaining to the level of quality of health care provided by various institutions—private and public hospitals, as well as those for veterans—and states any complications involved. It provides information on how to file a complaint, as well as information pertaining to Medicare coverage for health-care services.

(20) (C) To ensure patients are addressed directly

Such an omission might occur due to distractions, like the nurse focusing on the patient's most affected area, such as the location of an incision. The nurse's focus might also be on the patient's medications or treatment in general, or any other patient-related issues. Protocol dictates that the nurse should first greet the patient, make introductions, and then let the patient speak.

(21) (D) Training the nurses on how to communicate effectively

While patients require attention and empathy, sometimes nurses focus too much on designated tasks, leaving no room to communicate well with patients. It is advisable for nurses to converse with patients even as they work, as it increases patient satisfaction.

(22) (B) The health provider's colleagues

When colleagues get along well, patients benefit. This model also emphasizes the importance of having professionals provide care for a reasonable length of time because with continuity, trust between them and the patients tends to become stronger.

(23) (C) Hold a meeting with supervisors of all units to get their input

The reason it is good to consult with supervisors is that they often know the sectors where new RNs must be better prepared. It is also important to consult other members of staff about what they think might be improved in the orientation program.

(24) (A) To accept there is a problem and offer an apology for it

Note that acknowledging a shortcoming is different from accepting blame. If staff has been late in attending to a patient, you can say, "I apologize for the inconvenience you have been caused." Denying a problem can make a patient resentful.

(25) (D) Involving staff from every level and area of an organization

A partnership council can comprise staff from housekeeping, IT, nursing, and the laboratory. With such variety, the needs or challenges of the organization can be viewed from different perspectives.

(26) (B) Having a good understanding of your audience

That understanding helps determine the best verbal language and body language to use. Additional elements that are important in persuasive communication include anecdotes, pieces of information that are interesting, explaining your area of expertise, and providing information on how the service is meant to benefit an individual.

(27) (C) The topic and purpose

Although there should be a script that is followed, the health provider should not recite it verbatim when interacting with a patient. The script is meant to be a guide that ensures every important element is covered; the suitable words to use depend on the needs of every individual patient.

(28) (A) Identifying patients who can be safely discharged early

This could include cancellation of previously scheduled procedures, like any elective surgery. Additional beds can also be set up within the outpatient area and in clear hallways; it is faster than shifting patients to other rooms and cleaning those cleared rooms. There may also be a need to divert clients to different hospitals.

(29) (A) Text messages

Young patients may just ignore emails, and they may not bother opening unsolicited postal mail. Their main mode of communication is text messaging, and they are likely to read texts and respond to them. Text messaging is especially convenient when you want to remind a young patient of an appointment.

(30) (C) Spiral

A career is deemed linear when the individual rises up the career ladder progressively, and it is entrepreneurial or transient when the individual has the tendency to take up temporary jobs or practice privately. When a career is in a steady state, the individual gains experience over a long time, but that does not translate to added authority.

(31) (D) Engaging in false imprisonment

For the charge of false imprisonment to hold, the individual must have been physically restrained or denied exit, like when doors are locked and the individual does not have access to the keys. It can also be deemed false imprisonment if the person is made to believe he/she is not allowed to leave.

(32) (B) Offer flexible schedules and assignments

Such staff may be prepared to work for short hours or on a less strenuous work schedule. Some might be receptive to the idea of being retrained for a related job that is not as physically demanding as their present job.

(33) (C) Forming patient/family advisory councils

These councils comprise medical staff from varying departments as well as patients and family members. They result in a reasonably good understanding of the challenges the patients are facing and are able to provide better insight into what might be helpful to individual patients. These councils, nevertheless, are not authorized to take any action.

(34) (D) Multifactor productivity

Multifactor productivity is another term used to refer to total factor productivity. This reflects the total outputs that result from several traditional inputs.

(35) (A) Many different factors can have a positive or negative impact on productivity.

Factors such as staff competency, work methods, and established procedures all have the potential to negatively or positively affect productivity. You can have a positive impact on productivity by enhancing staff competency, applying improved procedures, and hiring competent management teams.

(36) (C) Content addressing their short-term learning needs

Adults are most motivated by content that addresses their short-term learning needs or goals. For example, nursing orientees are more interested in the procedures and policies of their new unit and less interested in the background of the health facility. This is because adults tend to focus on resolving an immediate problem.

(37) (C) The act became law in 2010.

In 2010, the Patient Protection and Affordable Care Act, known as Obamacare, was passed into law.

(38) (B) 1.32

To determine the asset/liability ratio, divide the total assets' value, which is $1,000,000,000 by the value of total liabilities, which is $654,639,098. Therefore, $1,000,000,000/$754,739,089 = 1.324. Round this to get 1.32.

(39) (B) Orientation is usually a process, not an event.

This process is usually systematic and well planned and continues even after the first orientation period is over. Orientation often goes on for months until the orientee is considered a fully competent worker in most or all areas of the job.

(40) (D) He should work with the staff to identify ways to reduce the need to work overtime.

Negative variances indicate that a facility or organization is spending more money than what it has budgeted, while positive variances indicate that the money spent is below the budgeted amount. To correct this negative variance, James should work with the staff to identify ways that may reduce the need for them to work overtime.

(41) (A) Job analysis, screening, sourcing, and selection

Job specification and job description are established in the job analysis stage, while the sourcing phase determines recruitment strategies. Screening entails analyzing the ability, skills, and knowledge of the applicants as per job requirements, while selection involves determining the candidate who is most qualified for the job.

(42) (D) It ensures that data collected is accurate and helps nurse executives make informed decisions.

Computerized accounting systems use spreadsheets, such as Excel, that are less prone to errors compared to paper accounting systems. This helps the organization make knowledgeable choices. The systems also allow data to be easily manipulated, which helps the organization perform complex analyses.

(43) (C) The philosophy, goals, and mission of the health facility

The goal of a selection process should be to identify the candidate who is most qualified for the job and who understands and is ready to adhere to the goals, mission, and philosophy of the medical facility. This document provides the right framework for conducting interviews that facilitate this goal.

(44) (C) It was founded in 1955 under the United States Department of Health and Human Services.

The Indian Health Service is a federally registered program that was established under the U.S. Department of Health and Human Services in 1995. Many Alaskan natives and Native Americans in the United States receive health services through this federally funded program.

(45) (C) An overqualified individual whose qualifications far exceed the job expectations

An overqualified candidate is an asset to an organization. Managers should not feel threatened by overqualified candidates and should instead view them as members who may benefit the organization.

(46) (D) Tell us a bit about your accomplishments and aspirations.

Open-ended questions give the interviewee an opportunity to give more details and information. A closed-ended question, on the other hand, can simply be answered using a "No" or a "Yes."

(47) (D) Outcome: Severity of any falls

An outcome-oriented performance improvement focus looks into the seriousness of a fall. Other measurements that are focused on outcomes include number of falls, satisfaction levels of patients, and patient compliance.

(48) (A) Fire extinguishers

All employees are required to know what to do in case of emergencies, such as fire. Training on how to properly use an extinguisher should be given to all new employees during orientation.

(49) (D) Gathering data, planning, coming up with a budget, negotiating or revising, and evaluating

The first step in a budgeting process involves the thorough collection of relevant data. The second step is to plan the budget according to the organization's objectives, mission, and priorities. Once the budget is planned, it is analyzed, negotiated, revised accordingly, and lastly, evaluated.

(50) (A) It is timely, complete, effective, and appropriate.

A successful orientation should be timely and effective, meaning that it should begin right after employment and achieve the desired outcome. It should also be complete and appropriate, meaning that it should completely address all the necessary aspects of the job and suit the employee's new role.

(51) (D) Operating budgets are used for patient care equipment with costs less than $1,000.

The main difference is that the operating budget deals with patient care equipment whose cost is less than $1,000, while the capital budget deals with equipment whose cost is more than $1,000.

(52) (B) Medicare prospective compensation

DRGs determine how much reimbursement Medicare is required to provide. It determines this figure based on a patient's needs, medical diagnosis, and the required procedures instead of considering the cost of services and the duration of stay at the facility. This makes it a prospective kind of compensation.

(53) (A) Unclear roles within empowered organizations

Many empowered organizations are characterized by autonomy or independent decision-making. This characteristic can easily cause role ambiguity, which may end up causing organizational conflict.

(54) (C) Indifference

Indifference is an indicator that the staff is rejecting or resisting the change. Other behavioral indicators include frustration, passive resistance, active resistance, and overt acceptance of the change paired with covert resistance. Reemergence and equilibrium, on the other hand, are positive indicators that the staff is accommodating the change.

(55) (B) Clarify the differences according to the individuals' goals and priorities

Frustration during a conflict is mainly caused by a difference in opinions and perspectives regarding beliefs and values relating to a certain issue. Clarifying these differences according to each party's goals and priorities is, therefore, the most ideal approach to use.

(56) (D) Catalyzing

Catalyzing is a mentorship technique used in professional development programs in which a mentor places his mentee in an unfamiliar and complex situation. The aim is to encourage new ways of reasoning and solving problems.

(57) (A) Failure to define the issue or problem accurately

The most crucial step in a problem-solving process is accurately identifying the problem. When a problem is poorly identified or defined, the problem-solving outcome is also poor, and the chances of having the problem recur increase.

(58) (A) Flowchart

Flowcharts are ideal for effectively identifying and analyzing the steps in complex processes. They illustrate the processes using directional arrows and sequential boxes and are especially ideal for groups, since flowcharts attempt to improve processes.

(59) (C) Mentees receive new and advanced techniques and perspectives.

Reverse mentorship is a type of mentorship in which an older mentee is coupled with a younger mentor whose skills or abilities are beneficial to the mentee. The benefit of this kind of mentoring is that the mentee has an opportunity to acquire new, advanced techniques and perspectives.

(60) (D) Conflict frequently reoccurs.

When a conflict keeps recurring in an organization, it may be an indication that the conflict cannot be solved using normal conflict-resolution interventions. Such conflicts occur when two opposing forces have negative and positive consequences that are equal in value.

(61) (D) Total quality management, quality management

Quality management was previously known as total quality management. Other terms that were previously used include quality assurance, quality control, continuous quality improvement, and total quality management. Today the new terms used are performance improvement, quality management, and quality improvement.

(62) (B) A man with a language barrier

A patient who cannot effectively communicate with a health-care giver is more prone to medical errors. Other types of patients who are at risk of medical errors include infants and patients with cognitive impairments, sensory disorders, psychiatric disorders, or developmental disorders.

(63) (C) The causes that are "not applicable" must also be explained.

To be deemed credible, the root-cause analysis must contain explanations for all the causes, including those that are indicated as being "not applicable." Every step under investigation should be carefully analyzed and the possible causes documented.

(64) (B) A flattened and decentralized organizational structure

A magnet hospital has a flattened and decentralized organizational structure. This is the performance improvement structure that replaced the hierarchical structure.

(65) (C) Fear of losing control

Some nursing managers and supervisors fear that if the nursing staff is empowered, then they stand to lose control or power over staff. Empowering the staff may be greatly beneficial to an organization, so this kind of fear hinders both self-development and the organization's development.

(66) (B) Consumers

The consumer, who is also the patient or the customer, is the main link among all the relationships that are found in a health-care setting. The needs, values, and views of the customer are the main determinants of how a health-care facility is run.

(67) (D) Using two unique resident identifiers

The usage of two unique resident identifiers is a National Patient Safety Goal for health-care settings. Other care goals included in the program relate to central line infections, pressure ulcers, and falls, among others.

(68) (C) They are created by many companies.

Many different companies are now producing CIS technology programs. There are several factors that an organization should consider when sourcing a CIS that suits its needs. These include the cost, how easy it is to use the program, and the capabilities of the program.

(69) (A) Class B

Class C extinguishers are used to extinguish electrical fires. Class A extinguishers are used for fires made from wood, mattresses, and paper, while Class B extinguishers are used for fires caused by oil or grease.

(70) (B) Problem-solving

This process seeks to eliminate the gap that lies between the current situation and the desired situation. Divergent thinking, empowerment, and decision-making are all different processes even though decision-making and divergent thinking are useful processes in problem-solving.

(71) (A) Optimizing

In decision-making, optimizing is the most time-consuming model, but it facilitates the most ideal decisions. The main objective of the optimizing model is to identify the most ideal solution after investigating all the costs, risks, and benefits of the alternative solutions.

(72) (D) Continuously

HIPAA requires health-care facilities to carry out continuous risk analysis as a way of strategically managing patient information technology. The risk analysis should include identifying security incidents and reviewing access tracking records.

(73) (D) Havelock's Six Phases of Planned Change

The first phases of Havelock's theory include developing relationships, diagnosing the problem, and actively acquiring the needed resources. The other phases of the theory are choosing solutions, gaining acceptance, and stabilizing change.

(74) (C) Collaborating, compromising, avoiding, competing, and accommodating

Collaborating, compromising, avoiding, competing, and accommodating are the five different modes used in conflict resolution.

(75) (B) Learning objectives

PowerPoint slides are ideal for learning purposes because they are used to briefly summarize key information points. Policies and narrative accounts, on the other hand, are too long for PowerPoint slides.

(76) (D) Move all the patients away from the windows and wait for further instructions

If a tornado watch alert is given, move all the patients away from the windows and wait for further instructions. Where possible, you may also move the patients to a lower floor in the building.

(77) (A) Nursing Informatics

The Nursing Informatics certification by the ANCC qualifies a nurse working in the information technology field. ANCC does not offer nursing technology, health information, or health technology certifications.

(78) (B) The Needlestick Safety and Prevention Act

This act requires employers to identify and utilize safe medical devices to ensure the safety of the staff who work in the facility. The law is meant to enhance safety in the workplace by reducing or eliminating accidents caused by sharp objects.

(79) (D) Determine the factors that are causing the procrastination

The first step is to identify the issues that lead to your procrastination. Deal with that particular area first, then move on to the other areas of the project.

(80) (C) Initiation, planning, implementing, monitoring, completion

The steps involved in project management are initiation, planning, implementing, monitoring, and completion. These steps may be likened to those of a problem-solving process that involves identifying the problem, choosing an option, implementing, and evaluating.

(81) (A) Solidifying of blood

Some of the engineering controls used to promote workplace safety include solidifying of blood and use of retractable scalpel blades and needleless systems.

(82) (B) Bioterrorism contingency plan

The military and its response teams are supposed to be a part of a health-care organization's bioterrorism contingency plan. Bioterrorism is an attack involving the intentional release of toxins, bacteria, or viruses into the environment with the intent of harming people.

(83) (D) They help in maintaining quality and reducing risk despite the constant changes in the external and internal environment.

The main purpose of having a contingency plan within a business is to maintain quality standards and reduce risk despite the constant changes in the external and internal environment. Effectiveness, timeliness, and efficiency are all features of quality.

(84) (D) Agreeing in principle and receiving criticism without turning defensive

Fogging is a communication technique that gives the manager room to be sincere about his/her stance without turning defensive. Even then, it is important to understand all important communication techniques so that you can choose the one suited for each circumstance. For example, fogging would not be appropriate in a situation involving someone giving aggressive criticism.

(85) (D) Cybernetic model

There are three phases in the cybernetic model: needs assessment, program implementation, and assessment of results. It is in the third phase where the objectives of the program are evaluated alongside the cost and the impact.

(86) (C) Do you have children? If so, how many?

It is unacceptable to ask about the candidate's children because this can be considered discriminatory on family grounds; the candidate can even sue if he/she is not hired. Instead, you can establish if the candidate would be available to work long hours by asking about the maximum number of hours he/she can work in a week.

(87) (D) Libel

Libel is correct, as it means the patient was defamed, and it legally amounts to an intentional tort. If the negative things had been only spoken, the charge would have been slander. Even if the nurses had written truths about the patient but the intention was to negatively influence the nature of health care provided, the charge would still be libel.

(88) (D) STD testing and STD treatment, excluding HIV

A registered nurse can also provide informed consent regarding treatment or a procedure that either a minor or an adult requires. As for contraceptives, just 26 of all US states permit a minor to accept such services. For abortion, only a handful of states permit a minor to give informed consent.

(89) (C) They diminish the patient's autonomy.

The term *paternalism* is used to indicate that the nurse is using his/her personal judgment to make a decision for the patient without taking into account what the patient's ideas are regarding his/her situation. However, even while respecting the patient's autonomy, the ultimate decision must be sound according to the nurse, as per the beneficence principle.

(90) (C) Primary nursing

The other three models of nursing care delivery are total patient care, team nursing, and functional nursing. In the first model, a patient is taken care of by a single nurse during the shift; in the second, an RN delegates tasks to members of a team taking care of a tiny group of patients.

(91) (A) Acuity level

The patient classification system (PCS) measures acuity levels regarding the extent and quantity of care some patient populations require. Nurse executives are instrumental in developing PCSs.

(92) (D) To determine Medicare reimbursements at a set fee

Diagnostic-related group (DRGs) amendments were made to the Social Security Act in 1983, and they included Medicare beneficiaries' prospective system of payment.

(93) (A) State level

The departments of health and environment at the state level deal with matters pertaining to the disposal of medical waste. The Environmental Protection

Agency used to be in charge, but its authority ceased in 1991 after the expiration of the Medical Waste Tracking Act.

(94) (D) Provide patients with a notice in written form concerning the right they have to make decisions pertaining to their treatment

This act is an amendment to 1990's Omnibus Budget Reconciliation Act. The written information should be given at the time the patient is admitted to the institution.

(95) (A) SWOT analysis

The focus of this analysis includes four major attributes, which are the strengths, weaknesses, opportunities, and probable threats. If these are addressed, it becomes easier to handle challenges and take advantage of available opportunities.

(96) (A) Zero-based budgeting (ZBB)

Every new financial period, expenditures must be justified beforehand under zero-based budgeting. While this method of budgeting takes a long time to complete, its results are usually both current and largely accurate.

(97) (B) The capital budget

Capital budgets address costs of assets that last for several years, such as computers, medical equipment, beds, buildings, etc.

(98) (C) Benchmarking

This can include generic, functional, global, or performance benchmarking. It also has levels, like internal, where the benchmarking is done within the institution, such as comparing the service delivery of different departments. Another level could be benchmarking against other industries.

(99) (A) Intervention

An example is having RNs delegate work to other nurses. When RNs do so, they remain accountable for the task and need to be certain that any assisting staff is adequately qualified to handle the task being allocated to them. Guidelines for delegation are provided by the American Nurses Association.

(100) (B) Receive the three-shot hepatitis B vaccine

It is within the right of such employees to reject the vaccine, but if they decline, this must be recorded in their respective health files. After staff members are exposed to patients, any evaluation deemed necessary is done at the expense of the employer.

(101) (A) Harriet Tubman

Harriet Tubman was not only known for working in hospitals with Clara during the war. She also freed more than 700 slaves.

(102) (C) Sojourner Truth

Truth is known for her nursing services to black soldiers and for her positive contribution to the fight for African Americans' civil rights.

(103) (A) Isabel Hampton Robb

As nurse superintendent and principal of the training school at John Hopkins Hospital, Isabel H. Robb was able to effect great changes that benefitted student nurses and women. This included encouraging the hospital to admit women to study medicine. Not only did Robb reduce student work hours, but she pushed for the implementation of licensure examinations.

(104) (A) Mary Breckinridge

Mary Breckinridge, who was trained at New York City's St. Luke's Hospital School of Nursing, was motivated to focus on the improvement of children's welfare by her loss of a daughter and a son.

(105) (D) Mildred Montag

Mildred Montag believed the associate degree would impact the education provided in nursing community colleges. She had a PhD and was the founder of the Adelphi College School of Nursing.

(106) (B) Lavinia Dock

Lavinia Dock belonged to the Women's Trade Union League. She is also remembered for publicly advocating for the right of women to have birth control.

(107) (B) Virginia Henderson

Virginia Henderson developed the theory that nurses need to enhance the independence of patients so they can make progress faster while still hospitalized.

(108) (A) Mary Mahoney

Mary Mahoney was born in Boston in 1845 and trained at New England Hospital. In 1879, she became the first woman of black descent to undergo full nursing training. She is in the Nursing Hall of Fame.

(109) (D) Hildegard Peplau

The theory Peplau developed includes the components of the person; the environment within the cultural context; health; and other processes of a human nature, like creativity and productivity.

(110) (C) Melinda Ann (Linda) Richards

Melinda Richards, popularly known as Linda, was the first American-trained nurse. She helped initiate several nursing schools in the United States and Japan.

(111) (B) Margaret Sanger

Margaret Sanger started the first clinic in the United States, based in Brooklyn, that provided birth-control services. She formed a committee to prepare relevant legislation, and in the 1950s she was president of the International Planned Parenthood Federation.

(112) (A) Lillian Wald

Not only was Ward a well-known nurse, but she also contributed to public health as an official. She was a social worker and an activist in the civil rights movement.

(113) (A) A cholera outbreak occurred in Ireland, where nurses from the Sisters of Mercy were selfless in helping patients.

Nuns of Irish descent developed a comprehensive nursing system that focused on stringent care in nursing.

(114) (C) Visiting the sick at home and later starting a hospital in Cincinnati

The sisters would visit the sick at home. Later, they visited them in the hospital when one was established in Cincinnati.

(115) (C) Boston

Linda Richards graduated in 1873 from Boston's New England Hospital.

(116) (A) Military nursing orders

Any of the military nursing orders were referred to as "Knight's Hospitaller." Its male nurses cared for the sick pilgrims coming into Jerusalem, along with those who were injured or poor. The orders worked under Jerusalem's Hospital of Saint John.

(117) (D) The Crimean War

Nightingale assembled a 38-nurse team to care for British war soldiers during the Crimean War.

(118) (C) The Nurse Reinvestment Act

The ANA supported the act that authorized many helpful provisions, which included programs for repaying loans, long-term training grants, and public service announcements encouraging people to choose nursing as a career.

(119) (A) During a public health emergency, covered entities may disclose protected medical information without the authorization of the individual.

Health-care providers have the authority to share information among themselves if doing so can help reduce the chances of the disease spreading. HIPAA rules also restrict an individual from accessing information of a medical nature if the person is involved in a clinical trial as long as that person agreed to such a restriction from the beginning.

(120) (B) Metanalysis

Metanalysis is used for the purpose of integrating the outcomes from different studies but on the same topic. This analysis helps identify patterns common in all the studies.

(121) (C) The board must have a member who has no affiliation with the institution.

Regulation of IRBs is done by the FDA and the Department of Health and Human Resources. Any institution that receives research funding from the federal government is required to have such a board, whose main role is to protect research participants' rights.

(122) (C) Managed-care companies on contract

An internal customer is a person working within the hospital who receives services from the hospital. Examples include doctors and health-care staff who render services from the hospital premises. External customers consume services from the hospital but are not under the hospital payroll like doctors are.

(123) (C) Involve the staff in the transition and hold a staff meeting to provide further information, even as you welcome any feedback

It is important to share the institution's goals with the staff, especially those bound to be impacted by the changes. It is also advisable to encourage open dialogue and make an effort to lessen staff concerns.

(124) (C) Collaboration

When conflict is well managed, an institution is bound to benefit. Some styles of conflict management include compromise, avoidance, accommodation, and collaboration. Force is another style of conflict resolution sometimes used. Avoidance, though nonconfrontational, does not often help in resolving conflict.

(125) (C) Employees should not be subjected to a minimum wage, since they are salaried.

The Fair Labor Standards Act is administered at the federal level by the Labor Department. Laws related to labor are established under this act, like those that stipulate compensation of overtime or what constitutes child labor. Employees are deemed exempt when they are salaried and hence not qualified for overtime.

(126) (B) Reporting all specified sentinel events

The policy's goals include improving care for patients, reducing the regularity of sentinel events, increasing knowledge pertaining to the events, and ensuring the public maintains its confidence in accredited organizations. Though a hospital is required to spell out what its sentinel events are, it does not have to report the events to the commission.

(127) (C) Fall of a patient that led to permanent and total loss of limb function

The policy spells out those sentinel events that are reviewable and those that are not. Reviewable events result in death that could not have been anticipated or in unanticipated permanent incapacitation. The Joint Commission carries out the review.

(128) (B) 1.0 mg

Having a trailing zero in a dosage, like 1.0 mg, or lacking a lead zero, like .1 mg, is viewed by the Joint Commission as a potential danger. The reason they are on the Do Not Use list is that one can confuse 1.0 for 10 or 0.1 for 1, which is a grave variation in medicine.

(129) (C) The actions of the nurse were directly connected to the injury the patient sustained.

Malpractice, as per the Joint Commission, is unethical behavior. It also encompasses an unreasonable skill deficiency on the part of a professional. There needs to be proof of the relationship linking a patient's injury to a nurse's behavior. The causality of it needs to be proven as substantial and not simply direct.

(130) (B) The subject signing informed consent

Per the Department of Health and Human Services' privacy rule, issued in 2003, information regarding a person's health should remain protected even as research findings are disclosed.

(131) (A) The state

De-identification allows information pertaining to someone's health, which is otherwise protected, to be disclosed under the HIPAA rule that addresses matters of research. There are 18 elements of a descriptive nature that require removal before disclosure can be made in order to keep a person's identity private.

(132) (B) Norming

At first, there were four Tuckman's stages, but they later expanded when a stage of adjourning was added. Forming is the initial stage, where a group is formed, and communication is initiated. The second stage is storming, and then norming follows, where the addressing of goals begins. The performing and adjourning stages then follow, in that order.

(133) (D) Legitimate power

The basis of legitimate power is the authority position that a leader holds within an organization. Power types that are an indication of followers' positive outlook toward their respective leaders include the "expert" as well as the "referent." Under these power types, followers go beyond compliance and manifest respect alongside commitment.

(134) (C) Lateral violence

Lateral violence can be in the form of sabotage, withholding of information, or nonverbal language like gestures. Newly hired nurses are the most common victims, and it is a difficult problem to solve, as the behavior is usually covert. Educating staff may be helpful, alongside adopting a no-tolerance policy in the institution.

(135) (A) Listeriosis

The requirement that infectious diseases be reported by laboratories and providers of health care in general is a stipulation of state laws and those of local authorities.

(136) (D) Office of the Inspector General

It is the role of the Office of the Inspector General to protect the DHHS's programs. Also, this office liaises with the Department of Justice and the FBI to detect fraud and prevent it.

(137) (D) Nursing hours for each patient day

The ANA developed nine secure staffing principles in 1998. When plans for staffing are being designed, one question that comes up is the nursing hours per patient days.

(138) (D) The nurse manager approving all new employees through the hospital's nurse executive

Decision-making is centralized when major elements of business are restricted to the topmost level of an organization's management. A good example is when the nurse manager uses a nurse executive to approve new-staff hiring. The process is relatively quick and communication is consistent, but employees are not accorded a chance to be creative.

(139) (C) All-or-nothing thinking

Another term for this cognitive distortion is black-and-white thinking, and people who apply it are usually perfectionists. They find it extremely hard to handle unreasonable demands. In this case, it is better for the nurse executive to address the issue of inadequate budgeting than to focus on the unit manager's inability to meet expectations.

(140) (C) It identifies the principles of ethics that serve as the basis for establishing the Health and Human Services' regulations meant to protect human subjects.

The Belmont Report was initially a compilation of principles and ethics guidelines meant to protect people used as research subjects. The principles of ethics included in the report are respect for the subjects, beneficence, and justice.

(141) (D) Reducing older workers' benefits in order to match younger workers' cost of benefits

The federal law that prohibits employment discrimination is enforced by the Equal Employment Opportunity Commission. Anyone basing remuneration on race, color, religion, gender, nationality, genetics, age or disability is breaking the law. As for the wage reduction, it may be permissible under certain circumstances.

(142) (C) To prevent disease and promote health for every American

The goal of the HP2020 program is to promote health while preventing disease. It has several objectives that pertain to people's health, including 42 areas of focus under which data is analyzed in the course of reviewing progress.

(143) (D) Employer's Liability Insurance

Not only does this insurance cover employers against their employees' negligence, but it also covers them against their failure to equip the employees with safe gear or a safe work environment. To cover liability for injury to third parties, the relevant insurance is public liability insurance.

(144) (D) Part C

As per Part C, the part with Medicare Advantage plans, participants under Medicare benefit from health care through private health insurance. A participant can benefit from Part C only if he/she already has Parts A and B of Medicare.

(145) (C) Air embolism

Illnesses not covered under the Deficit Reduction Act's Section 5001(C) include those that a patient develops while hospitalized. These include air embolisms, receiving incompatible blood, having a foreign object forgotten in the body during surgery, and urinary tract infections from the use of catheters and other items.

(146) (B) Data sheets pertaining to safety issues and a full list of dangerous chemicals

An Exposure Control Plan includes many items, among them determining that an employee has actually been exposed, implementing methods of controlling exposure, documentation pertaining to hepatitis B vaccinations, evaluation after exposure, training of employees, recordkeeping, and procedures that evaluate events that lead to exposure.

(147) (C) Failure mode and effects analysis

The failure mode and effects analysis serves as a method for identifying potential modes or processes of failure. Once identified, a proper analysis is carried out and recommendations are made on the best action to take.

(148) (B) Pareto chart

The 80/20 rule is the Pareto principle that an economist from Italy created. Although he meant it to be a measure of how uneven wealth distribution was, it proved useful in other areas. The Pareto chart helps in maintaining a focus on causes and factors of utmost importance, according them priority.

(149) (B) A Gantt is a form of bar chart, while a PERT chart is a form of flowchart.

A Gantt chart, which is a linear bar chart, is used in the display of a project's schedule. Meanwhile, PERT flowcharts target the relationships among different activities, which are normally large, complex projects.

(150) (C) National Committee for Quality Assurance

The NCQA is a nonprofit organization that promotes quality health care. This organization has many programs, including accreditation of health plans, doctors, medical-based groups, and others.

Test 2: Questions

(1) Which of the following is an indicator of quality that is nursing-sensitive?

(A) Readmission rate of patients

(B) The cost of care

(C) Patient acuity classification

(D) The mix of skills among the nursing staff

(2) During a root-cause analysis, the peer review process determined that one nurse was not providing the same level of care as other practitioners. What recommendation should a nurse executive give in a situation like this?

(A) The individual should be fired.

(B) The individual should be placed on mandatory leave.

(C) The individual should get additional training and education.

(D) The individual should receive mentorship and support.

(3) Which of the following actions, according to Lewin/Schein's Change Theory, may be involved in the theory's initial stage, referred to as "unfreezing"?

(A) Identifying the needed changes

(B) Overriding defensive actions

(C) Changing perceptions of the individual and relationships

(D) Learning-related and survival-related anxiety

(4) What should be the first step in emergency planning?

(A) Assessing cost

(B) Reviewing past emergencies

(C) Analyzing vulnerability to hazards

(D) Surveying the policies of other institutions

(5) What step should an organization take if overall staff turnover exceeds 6 percent, which is the institution's benchmark?

(A) Develop a retention strategy

(B) Analyze this rate based on the class the job falls under

(C) Compare salaries by carrying out a study

(D) Survey the staff based on job satisfaction

(6) A census done in the surgical unit and oncology unit determined that there was a wide fluctuation between the two units, and this was the likely cause of understaffing and overstaffing. What is the ideal solution for such a situation?

(A) Laying off some staff members

(B) Cross-training staff

(C) Reassigning staff to different units

(D) Temporarily assigning staff to the understaffed unit

(7) What should be the first step in engaging patients when the aim is to increase patient engagement per the Patient Activation Measure?

(A) Being persistent in stressful times

(B) Having the resources or ability to facilitate action

(C) Acknowledging the important role that patients play

(D) Improving health by taking action

(8) What does the "platinum rule," the one that helps improve relationships between nurses and physicians, state?

(A) You should treat all alike.

(B) You should treat each person differently.

(C) You should treat people the way they prefer to be treated.

(D) You should treat people as you would like to be treated.

(9) What percentage of employees must first sign the union authorization card in order for their organization to voluntarily recognize that union as the employees' representative agent?

(A) 20 percent

(B) 30 percent

(C) 40 percent

(D) 50 percent

(10) Which two elements are considered forces of change, according to Lewin's Force Field model?

(A) Restraining and driving

(B) Effort and time

(C) Benefits and costs

(D) Administration and staff

(11) Which of the following change strategies characterizes the normative re-educative approach?

(A) Using data as a way of influencing others

(B) Using power as a way of forcing change

(C) Setting arbitrary standards

(D) Focusing on enhancing relations with others

(12) What problems are best solved using the Plan-Do-Study-Act method of quality improvement?

(A) Problems of a specific nature

(B) Organization-wide problems

(C) All problems

(D) Interdisciplinary problems

(13) What is the major use of training output estimation?

(A) Determining whether additional training is needed

(B) Estimating training-related outcomes

(C) Estimating practitioner supply in the health-care sector

(D) Evaluating how training is clinically applied

(14) What action should you take in verifying that new hires have the correct credentials and licenses?

(A) Contact their previous employers

(B) Ask the individuals to provide detailed information

(C) Conduct verifications from the primary sources

(D) Request that the individuals present their credentials and licenses

(15) Which of the following shows the four main criteria for privileging and credentialing?

(A) Necessity, performance ability, licensure, and recommendation

(B) Licensure, education, recommendation, and necessity

(C) Education, performance ability, competence, and licensure

(D) Education, recommendation, experience, and licensure

(16) What step must a nurse executive first take before instituting SBAR for use in an organization?

(A) Ask the staff to do some research on SBAR

(B) Carry out a staff survey

(C) Mandate an implementation date

(D) Provide guidelines and training

(17) Which of the following shows the four elements of quality measure present in a pay-for-performance program?

(A) Performance, costs, patient experience, and outcomes

(B) Costs, outcomes, best practices, and timeliness

(C) Performance, outcome, structure/technology, and patient experience

(D) Outcomes, patient experience, timeliness, and costs

(18) Which of the following is considered output, per the general systems theory?

(A) Facts

(B) Praise

(C) Lived experience

(D) Altered behavior

(19) A nurse executive proposed changes, and nobody verbally opposed them. An anonymous survey was then carried out on the matters, and the findings indicated there was widespread opposition to the changes. What kind of power does this particular nurse executive exercise?

(A) Legitimate power

(B) Expert power

(C) Coercive power

(D) Informative power

(20) What should follow after shortlisting potential vendors for an upgrade of services and equipment?

(A) Requesting a quotation

(B) Developing a business plan

(C) Developing a budget allowance

(D) Requesting a proposal

(21) If the plan is to change the skill mix and have fewer RNs so as to save on cost and alleviate the nurse shortage, what should be the first step?

(A) Determine tasks that only RNs should handle

(B) Determine tasks that non-RNs can handle

(C) Carry out a survey to determine the wages for the different groups of staff

(D) Calculate how much of a reduction in RNs is needed to achieve the cost-reduction target

(22) A hospital institutes a fair culture that encourages staff to report any unsafe practices or incidences in the facility. What is the hospital likely to do when a nurse fails to read a medication order correctly and administers the wrong dosage to her patient?

(A) Fire the nurse for incompetence

(B) Place the nurse on probation

(C) Console and support the nurse

(D) Provide further training to the nurse

(23) What is the next step after implementing evidence-based changes?

(A) Assess the costs

(B) Measure outcomes

(C) Punish those who are not compliant

(D) Survey the staff

(24) What can a hospital do to improve retention when turnover rate is high and the hospital is struggling to recruit staff?

(A) Provide ladders for career growth

(B) Provide on-site childcare

(C) Provide employee lounges

(D) Provide educational benefits

(25) Who coordinates care for at-risk patients in a transitional care model?

(A) A team of caregivers

(B) A family physician

(C) An advanced practice nurse

(D) A family member who is trained in caregiving

(26) When calculating employment costs, which is the sum of salaries and benefits, what percentage do benefits approximately account for in the total cost?

(A) 10 percent

(B) 20 percent

(C) 30 percent

(D) 40 percent

(27) The yearly employee cost of staff meant to work with a new machine is valued at $100,000. Using the new machine, 15 percent of production time will increase efficiency by approximately 30 percent, and that will result in a $4,500 productivity advantage for the machine that cost $90,000. Estimating ROI, how long will it take for the machine to fully pay for its cost?

(A) 9 months

(B) 15 months

(C) 20 months

(D) 30 months

(28) Which of the following leadership styles are linked to situational leadership?

(A) Selling and telling, delegating, and participating

(B) Norming and forming, performing, and storming

(C) Conflicting and separating, asserting, and confronting

(D) Trust and self-disclosure, feedback, and listening

(29) Which type of analysis uses the cost of full-time staff and cost of overtime to determine savings?

(A) Cost-effective analysis

(B) Cost-benefit analysis

(C) Efficacy study

(D) Cost-utility analysis

(30) What should be done first when planning to offer staff members the opportunity to continue learning?

(A) Objectives should be defined.

(B) A survey on staff preferences should be conducted.

(C) A pilot group should be selected.

(D) A needs assessment should be conducted.

(31) Which patient assessment must an inpatient rehabilitation center submit in order to receive compensation from Medicaid and Medicare?

(A) MDS

(B) OASIS

(C) IRF-OASIS

(D) IRF-PAI

(32) Nurse executives who do not hire nurses in their twenties because they believe that such nurses will require family leave at some point for the sake of having a family are said to be discriminative. What is such discrimination called?

(A) Illegal discrimination

(B) Statistical discrimination

(C) Retaliation

(D) Gender discrimination

(33) What method of reporting would assure staff members that there will be no repercussions for internal whistleblowing and that the identity of whistleblowers will remain anonymous?

(A) Reporting in person

(B) Reporting via telephone

(C) Using several methods

(D) Reporting in writing

(34) A nurse executive is responsible for directing the hospital's nursing department, which has a total of 450 employees. Among these, 350 are licensed nurses, 30 are supervisors directly reporting to department heads, 60 are support staff, and 10 are heads of departments directly reporting to the nurse executive. How many people does the nurse executive control?

(A) 410

(B) 40

(C) 10

(D) 450

(35) What approach can a hospital employ to attract patients, even with a low marketing budget?

(A) Brand marketing

(B) Alliance marketing

(C) Above-the-line mass marketing

(D) Targeted marketing

(36) Based on Kotter and Cohen's theory, what is the first action that should be taken to bring about change?

(A) Build a team that can guide change

(B) Create a sense of urgency

(C) Communicate the importance of change

(D) Remove barriers that hinder change

(37) Which of the following methods is most likely to produce the ideal equitable measure for performance appraisals?

(A) Graphic rating

(B) Forced ranking

(C) Self-appraisal

(D) Behaviorally anchored rating scale

(38) What are staff nurses who work 20 hours in a week throughout the year referred to as in staffing terms?

(A) 0.2 FTE

(B) 0.5 FTE

(C) 2.0 FTE

(D) 1.0 FTE

(39) What is a requirement when an organization is implementing an affirmative action plan?

(A) Establishing the quota system for hiring

(B) Providing unbiased hiring opportunities so that all qualified candidates are considered

(C) Justifying the current hiring processes and practices

(D) Outlining steps for retaining minority staff members

(40) Which of the following is not a type of bargaining used in negotiation processes?

(A) Integrative bargaining

(B) Mixed bargaining

(C) Distributive bargaining

(D) Collaborative bargaining

(41) What does it mean to say that an article has gone through a double-blind review after being submitted by the writer?

(A) The identity of the writer was hidden from the reviewer.

(B) Neither the reviewer nor the writer knew the identity of the other.

(C) The identity of the reviewer was hidden from the writer.

(D) A software program was used to review the article.

(42) According to hospital 501(r) requirements, after what period should a nonprofit hospital carry out a community health needs assessment?

(A) One year

(B) Two years

(C) Three years

(D) Five years

(43) Which of the following internet sites provides consumers with information on the quality of doctors, hospitals, and dentists within any given area and matches profiles according to the criteria used in the search?

(A) RateMDs

(B) Hospital Compare

(C) WebMD

(D) Healthgrades

(44) Which of the following options shows the most crucial element in a disaster/emergency preparedness plan?

(A) A clearly outlined chain of command

(B) Established transfer protocols

(C) Availability of ready information and practice drills

(D) Triage protocols meant for dealing with injuries

(45) Which factors should be primarily considered when collecting data on clinical outcomes?

(A) Patient diagnosis and cost of care

(B) The vision and mission statement of the organization

(C) The requirements mandated for reporting and the population of patients

(D) Complications and duration of stay

(46) The decision-making method that considers the worst-case scenario is most encouraged when making ________ type of decisions.

(A) Personnel

(B) Everyday

(C) Financial

(D) Risky

(47) Provision one of the ANA Code of Ethics requires that all nurses respect their patients' rights. How should a nurse respond when a patient makes self-destructive or risky decisions?

(A) Remain silent as a way of respecting the patient's rights

(B) Express concerns while remaining supportive

(C) Address the worrying behavior and provide resources

(D) Point out the problems and criticize the behavior of the patient

(48) What system allows a physician from one hospital to access a patient's information from another hospital?

(A) CPOE

(B) EHR

(C) HIE

(D) CDSS

(49) Which of the following is the main protection accorded in the Patient's Bill of Rights of the Affordable Care Act?

(A) The right to choose a preferred physician

(B) Insurance coverage for preexisting health conditions

(C) Extension of insurance coverage for dependents up to age 21

(D) Limiting deductible charges by insurance companies

(50) Hospitals that attend to more than 10 patients in a day are required to give a quarterly report in compliance with ORYX®. How many electronic clinical quality measures must be reported by such hospitals?

(A) Five

(B) Six

(C) Nine

(D) Thirteen

(51) What are the criteria used in classifying accountability measures?

(A) Education, readiness, interventions, and complications

(B) Interventions, evidence, complications, and results

(C) Plan, study, do, and act

(D) Proximity and research, as well as adverse effects and accuracy

(52) What are nurse executives who promote pervasive leadership likely to do?

(A) Encourage others to make decisions

(B) Constantly check on subordinates

(C) Form a multi-tiered hierarchical system

(D) Take responsibility for every decision made

(53) A nurse executive wants to render additional services to an older population of patients at the hospital. The board of directors is supportive of the initiative but is not willing to fund the initiative. What should the nurse executive do?

(A) Look for any opportunities to get grants

(B) Gather additional data to present to the board

(C) Present a written protest to the board

(D) Ask the members of the community to pressure the board

(54) Several nurses are interested in carrying out research on evidence-based practices, but they do not have enough time to do so. What is the best advice that the nurse executive can give these nurses?

(A) Ask the staff members for time

(B) Form a journal club

(C) Carry out the research when there is not much to do during duty

(D) Use their paid time off to research

(55) Which principle in appreciative inquiry suggests that the actions of a person are influenced by his/her beliefs?

(A) The constructionist principle

(B) The anticipatory principle

(C) The positive principle

(D) The principle of simultaneity

(56) Which of the following statements is true about clinical research that is carried out using stored biospecimens with no identification?

(A) The research needs informed consent.

(B) The research is subject to Common Rule.

(C) Informed consent is not necessary.

(D) The research should be approved by IRB.

(57) What are the three Ps that facilitate successful consumer education?

(A) Practitioner, physician, and patient

(B) Priority, performance, and philosophy

(C) Persistence, permission, and performance

(D) Preparation, provision, and population

(58) What is the main element that enables clinical staff to establish evidence-based practice?

(A) Coercion

(B) Mentoring

(C) Reward systems

(D) Data or information

(59) Which of the following options is among the several phases Peplau's Interpersonal Relations Model of Nursing suggests nurse-patient relationships go through?

(A) Resolution of problems

(B) Problem evaluation

(C) Patient recovery

(D) Nurse-patient collaboration

(60) Major changes are expected to happen in a hospital when switching to the integrated CPOE, EHR, and CDSS. Which implementation method is most likely to cause the least disruption?

(A) Pilot study

(B) Big-bang implementation

(C) Gradual testing of changes

(D) Phased implementation

(61) What is the general goal of the Accelerated Rapid-Cycle Change approach?

(A) To come up with strategies that encourage behavioral health changes

(B) To respond to rapid change in a gradual manner

(C) To modify methods in order to increase the speed of response

(D) To focus on the importance of collaboration

(62) Who leads patient-centered medical homes?

(A) Therapists

(B) Case managers

(C) Nurse practitioners

(D) Personal physicians

(63) What state is a nurse likely to be in if he/she constantly licks his/her lips and rubs his/her hands together?

(A) A distracted state

(B) An angry state

(C) A nervous state

(D) A depressed state

(64) Which is the most suitable graphic display tool for showing age distribution data on a chart?

(A) A digital dashboard

(B) A scattergram

(C) A balanced scorecard

(D) A pie chart

(65) How can the steps of a process be adapted as a way of improving workflow?

(A) Increase them

(B) Combine them

(C) Eliminate them

(D) Use alternate paths

(66) What should an executive nurse focus on when using the leadership rounding tool to lead staff?

(A) Supervising staff

(B) Establishing rapport

(C) Inspecting units

(D) Identifying key stakeholders

(67) A nurse met with the unit supervisor and stated, “I see you have again used the most ideal solution to solve the problem.” What communication style was the nurse using?

(A) Assertive style

(B) Aggressive style

(C) Passive-aggressive style

(D) Persuasive style

(68) Which statement is true regarding patients assigned to any Accountable Care Organization through Medicare?

(A) Some of the patients’ information on their health is shared by various ACO providers among themselves.

(B) The patients can see only a specific physician who is assigned to them, and not their own physician of choice.

(C) Patients are allowed to participate in an HMO and an ACO at the same time.

(D) Patients can have their Medicare benefits changed once they are in the ACO.

(69) Which of the following is a socioeconomic indicator that may raise alarm and call for more screening in a patient’s case management?

(A) Resides in a low-income area

(B) Lacks the ability to drive

(C) Divorced with an adult child

(D) Admitted from a homeless shelter

(70) Which aspect of emotional intelligence does a nurse exhibit if he/she understands other people's feelings and understands why they are inclined to certain desires and needs?

(A) Empathy

(B) Self-awareness

(C) Social skills

(D) Motivation

(71) A nurse was concerned about the rising number of layoffs in her unit and shared these sentiments with her fellow nurse, who responded by saying, "You are afraid that you may also lose your job." What was the respondent practicing?

(A) Exploring

(B) Paraphrasing

(C) Reflecting

(D) Summarizing

(72) What should the nurse executive do when asked by the board of directors to add subordinate evaluations into the yearly performance review?

(A) Personally pick out subordinate evaluators

(B) Request that the reviews be signed by subordinates

(C) Suggest that the evaluations remain anonymous

(D) Inform the board of the potential bias that a subordinate evaluation may cause

(73) When a nurse executive makes eye contact, nods her head and asks questions as a subordinate is talking, what does that imply?

(A) She agrees with what the speaker is saying.

(B) She respects the suggestions given by the speaker.

(C) She is just appeasing the speaker.

(D) She will follow what the speaker is suggesting.

(74) Which of the following statements shows the use of a normative re-educative strategy used to manage changes?

(A) Providing figures and facts from research that support the changes

(B) Using authority to ensure that the staff adheres to the changes

(C) Using punishment and rewards to promote the changes

(D) Encouraging staff to identify any problems and come up with solutions

(75) What does change in a single area do, according to the STAR model of change?

(A) It results in unsuccessful change.

(B) It promotes accommodation of change.

(C) It triggers change in other areas.

(D) It causes unsuspected outcomes.

(76) Which factor must a nurse executive first explain to staff before initiating changes affecting procedures and processes?

(A) The learning curve

(B) The reason for the impending changes

(C) The time frame within which the change will be implemented

(D) The cost-effectiveness of the change

(77) What is the first factor that a nurse executive needs to consider before instituting telehealth programs for patients who are primarily covered under the original Medicare stipulations?

(A) The need for more staff and staff training

(B) How much the program would cost

(C) The impact that the program would have on inpatient services

(D) The geographical location of the population that is targeted

(78) What assessment may be suitably done by making use of small-area analysis?

(A) Mortality rates in hospitals all over the state

(B) The impact that reducing Medicaid would have on the entire state

(C) Morbidity rates in different states

(D) The rate of individual health facility utilization in the city

(79) According to Von Bertalanffy's system theory, which system element comprises actions that have the capacity to transform the input?

(A) Feedback

(B) Throughput

(C) Evaluation

(D) Output

(80) Under the Family and Medical Leave Act, how many weeks of leave is Kendra eligible for in one year so she can take care of her husband, who is an army officer recovering from injuries suffered while in the line of duty?

(A) 48 workweeks

(B) 10 workweeks

(C) 26 workweeks

(D) 12 workweeks

(81) What does Lean Six Sigma focus on as a method of process enhancement?

(A) Strategic goals

(B) Near-term goals

(C) Individual projects

(D) Individual staff members

(82) What do conformance costs represent in cost analysis?

(A) All necessary costs, such as processes, services, material, equipment, staff, and time costs

(B) Shared costs, like infrastructure costs

(C) Costs incurred due to errors, defects, and failures, including malpractice and duplication of services

(D) Costs incurred from products or services used to prevent errors or failures, such as evaluation and monitoring

(83) Which of the following is a legal term used in reference to the failure of an entity to perform its duties per set practice standards?

(A) Duty

(B) Breach

(C) Harm

(D) Causation

(84) In determining proof of negligence linked to malpractice, what does risk management term the act of intentionally providing substandard care while disregarding a patient's security and safety?

(A) Comparative negligence

(B) Contributory negligence

(C) Negligent conduct

(D) Gross negligence

(85) Which type of analysis is used in determining monetary savings from a planned intervention?

(A) Cost-utility analysis

(B) Cost-benefit analysis

(C) Efficacy analysis

(D) Cost-effective analysis

(86) Which of the following statements is true regarding Medicare Advantage?

(A) It is a supplemental insurance plan.

(B) It is an optional plan that Medicare provides.

(C) It is a plan that is authorized by Medicare and administered by private insurance firms.

(D) It is a type of medical assistance offered to Medicare recipients.

(87) Which of the following elements shows an organization's commitment to its strategic planning?

(A) Its vision statement

(B) Its objectives

(C) Its mission statement

(D) Its goals

(88) Which of the following actions meaningfully contributes to creating a healthy work environment?

(A) Providing an annual salary increase to staff

(B) Providing a salary increase and certification

(C) Congratulating a staff member for demonstrating exemplary skills in nursing that prevented an accident from occurring

(D) Praising the staff to the board of directors

(89) When developing a risk management plan, what should be the main focus of a statement of purpose?

(A) Clients' safety

(B) The program's scope

(C) Decreased liability

(D) Reduced financial risk

(90) Which governmental agency determines the Bloodborne Pathogens Standards?

(A) CDC

(B) OSHA

(C) EPA

(D) FDA

(91) Which area does the Continuous Quality Improvement model mainly focus on?

(A) The clients

(B) The administrative personnel

(C) The staff

(D) The organization and its processes

(92) After discharge, how soon should the data from the Inpatient Rehabilitation Facility's Patient Assessment Instrument on the Medicare Part C (Medicare Advantage) or Medicare Part A fee-for-service be sent to the CMS National Assessment Collection Database?

(A) Within 72 hours

(B) Within 7 days

(C) Within 27 days

(D) Within 17 days

(93) When was the first dispensary opened in Philadelphia to offer free care to patients, treat war injuries, and provide smallpox vaccines?

(A) During the Gulf War

(B) During the American Revolution

(C) During WWII

(D) During the Cold War

(94) Which of the following people were nurses whose contribution during the American Civil War was noted by the public?

(A) Beatrix Hamburg and Virginia Apgar

(B) Clara Barton and Sojourner Truth

(C) Dorothy Horstmann and Florence Nightingale

(D) Florence Wald and Phyllis Bodel

(95) When did Isabel Robb design a plan to ensure proper management of nurses?

(A) During the Cambodian War

(B) During the Cold War

(C) During the Korean War

(D) During the Spanish-American War

(96) As WWI raged, demand for more nurses increased, some being trained at the Army School of Nursing. What characteristics were required of these nurses?

(A) They had to be medium height and soft-spoken.

(B) They had to be well-behaved and not married.

(C) They had to be over 30 years old and authoritative.

(D) They had to be tall and soft-spoken.

(97) What was accomplished by the 1943 Bolton Act that was sponsored by Frances P. Bolton?

(A) It was responsible for the creation of the Nurse Cadet Corps in the United States.

(B) It made it possible for the first time for soldiers to attend to their injured colleagues.

(C) It succeeded in getting Congress to allocate money to cover the treatment of injured soldiers.

(D) It banned retired soldiers from joining politics.

(98) During the Gulf War, what did nurses primarily focus on?

(A) Triaging injured soldiers at every treatment stage

(B) Reaching the injured soldiers' families

(C) Ensuring the soldiers were fed a balanced diet

(D) There were no US nurses in the Gulf War

(99) What is the name of the international body that deals with nurses' welfare, both of an economic and social nature?

(A) ICN

(B) WHO

(C) UN

(D) ILO

(100) Which is the governing body that employs collective bargaining, professional advancement, and legislation to address the issues affecting registered nurses in the United States?

(A) The World Health Organization

(B) The American Nurses Credentialing Center

(C) The American Nurses Association

(D) The Red Cross

(101) Which organization deals directly with matters pertaining to the enhancement of nurses' education?

(A) The Commission on Collegiate Nursing Education

(B) The American Association of Colleges of Nursing

(C) The American Nurses Credentialing Center

(D) The American Academy of Nursing

(102) Which organization is in charge of accreditation for nurses in the United States?

(A) The Commission on Collegiate Nursing Education

(B) The American Nurses Credentialing Center

(C) The American Nurses Association

(D) The International Labor Organization

(103) Which organization licenses the various relevant state bodies to work together in matters of board formation, setting and monitoring exams, and licensing of nurses?

(A) The American Hospital Association

(B) The National Council of State Boards of Nursing

(C) The Department of Health and Human Services

(D) American Public Health Association

(104) What is the largest worldwide organization that honors exemplary performance standards of nursing?

(A) The World Health Organization

(B) International Labor Organization

(C) Sigma Theta Tau International

(D) The United Nations

(105) Which of the following options is not among the roles of the National Student Nurses Association?

(A) Mentoring students as they prepare for licensure

(B) Advocating for accessibility to health-care services

(C) Putting pressure on employers to pay high salaries to nurses

(D) Advocating for and contributing to the advancement of the education of nurses

(106) Which of the following is not part of the role of the National Organization for Associate Degree Nursing?

(A) Creating associate degree certification exams

(B) Reinforcing the associate degree's value

(C) Endorsing graduates with the nursing associate degree

(D) Mentoring students in high school who would like to acquire a nursing associate degree later

(107) The American Organization of Nurse Executives is a subsidiary of which organization?

(A) AHA

(B) WHO

(C) ICN

(D) ANCC

(108) Which of the following organizations ensures terminologies and definitions used in the field of nursing for diagnosis are uniform?

(A) WHO

(B) NANDA-International

(C) CDC

(D) FDA

(109) Which of the following is characterized by low expenses and plenty of information pertaining to health?

(A) Diagnostic services

(B) Curative services

(C) Therapeutic services

(D) Preventative services

(110) Which of the following is not a factor to be considered in rationing of health care?

(A) Suitability of rationing

(B) Level of rationing

(C) Age of the patient

(D) Transparency in rationing

(111) Which of the following is not true of an HMO in the United States?

(A) It releases funds in advance when there is an insured patient in need of health-care services.

(B) It consists of several medical insurance providers.

(C) It accepts a regular fee, monthly or yearly, for the insurance coverage provided.

(D) Its premiums are normally lower than those of other insurance plans.

(112) Which of the following is not true of community-based nursing care?

(A) The nurse needs to understand the patient as well as the patient's family.

(B) The nurse needs to understand the patient as well as the patient's community.

(C) The nurse providing community-based care needs to be a relative of the patient.

(D) Community-based nursing can be either short-term or long-term.

(113) Which of the following is not a characteristic of managed care plans?

(A) They have insurance contracts with health-care providers.

(B) The more flexible a managed care plan is, the more expensive it is.

(C) The amount the managed care pays for a patient depends on what other plans pay for similar services.

(D) HMOs constitute a type of managed-care plan.

(114) Which of the following does not constitute a feature of capitation in health care?

(A) The doctor providing primary care is paid a set amount of money per patient for a set period.

(B) Under capitation, the PCP is paid by the state government.

(C) Capitation is under a contract with an HMO.

(D) The other party involved in capitation is the IPA.

(115) Which of the following statements regarding a wearable monitor is incorrect?

(A) It can be implanted in the patient.

(B) It monitors the patient's physiological parameters.

(C) It is designed to monitor the patient's kidney function.

(D) It normally has a bedside monitor as one of its components.

(116) Which of the following is not a method of subcutaneously delivering insulin?

(A) Vial

(B) Arm

(C) Pen

(D) Pump

(117) Which of the following is not a health organization category?

(A) Tertiary

(B) Primary

(C) Nursery

(D) Secondary

(118) What is an SSU in the context of a health-care institution?

(A) A ward where patients with special needs are admitted

(B) A ward that admits patients for a short period; sometimes for just 48 hours

(C) A hospital that specializes in providing secondary health care

(D) A hospital that specializes in surgery

(119) What is not true of an acute-care hospital?

(A) It provides health-care services on a 24-hour basis.

(B) It has the capacity to cater to two or more patients at once.

(C) It has the capacity to diagnose and treat illnesses and injuries.

(D) It is not licensed to handle obstetric cases.

(120) Which of the following is not true of long-term-care?

(A) It lasts for more than 30 days.

(B) It is limited to providing medicines and any necessary injections.

(C) It includes treatment of chronic illnesses.

(D) It addresses a patient's medical and nonmedical needs.

(121) What does the term *acuity* mean?

(A) The nurse's level of accuracy in treating patients

(B) The intensity of care a patient requires

(C) The cuteness of a newborn

(D) The severity of an injury

(122) Which of the following statements is incorrect about subacute care?

(A) Patients who need it are normally not very ill.

(B) Patients who need it are never hospitalized.

(C) Patients who need it can be treated as outpatients.

(D) Patients who need it are sometimes unable to function independently.

(123) What is the term given to health care that involves observing, assessing, and treating the patient while being fully responsible for the patient's care as a registered nurse?

(A) Medicare

(B) Acute care

(C) Skilled nursing care

(D) Nursing diagnosis

(124) Which of the following activities fall under ADLs?

(A) Exercising or walking on a treadmill for physical fitness

(B) Bathing and selecting suitable clothes to wear for the day

(C) Baking a birthday cake and icing it

(D) Breaking a coconut and blending it into a smoothie

(125) Which of the following is not part of hospice care?

(A) Providing medical care to the patient

(B) Taking the patient to visit as many friends as possible before dying

(C) Providing spiritual support to the patient's family members

(D) Providing spiritual support to the patient

(126) What is the purpose of rehab care?

(A) To help patients learn how to avoid future dangers to their health

(B) To help patients assess their physical capacity in comparison to other patients

(C) To help patients regain their health and function as normally as possible

(D) To help patients learn new skills and become better than they were before their illness

(127) Which of the following represents an instance when patients are released as soon as they are treated?

(A) When patients have no medical insurance

(B) When patients are receiving ambulatory care

(C) When health care is home-based

(D) When care is given in a nursing home

(128) What is not true of home health care?

(A) Family members play an important role in ensuring the individual's health does not deteriorate.

(B) Therapy services can also be provided under home health care.

(C) Nurses can make visits to dress the wounds of patients under home health care.

(D) Nurses cannot provide intravenous services to patients under home health care.

(129) Which of the following statements is incorrect?

(A) Federal hospitals treat specific categories of patients.

(B) Community hospitals are run by the federal government.

(C) Non-federal psychiatric care hospitals are mostly privately owned.

(D) Most physicians and nurses are trained in community hospitals.

(130) Which of the following is not specific to a tertiary care hospital?

(A) Trauma center

(B) Immunology center

(C) Oncology unit

(D) Burn center

(131) What is true of specialty hospitals?

(A) They charge different fees from other hospitals.

(B) They treat all types of diseases and perform all types of surgeries.

(C) The doctors in these hospitals offer free services.

(D) They specialize in providing specific types of health care.

(132) Which of the following is not true of the US Department of Health and Human Services?

(A) It fosters advancement in medicine and public health.

(B) It has different divisions under it, including the CDC, CMS, FDA, and others.

(C) It issues approval for health-care institutions.

(D) It is in charge of regulating health-care insurance coverage.

(133) Which of the following is not true of JCAHO?

(A) It is the sole body charged with accreditation of health-care institutions.

(B) All accreditation-related costs are paid by the organization seeking accreditation.

(C) It is within the purview of JCAHO to determine why infections occur in health-care institutions.

(D) More than 20,000 US health-care institutions have been accredited by JCAHO.

(134) Which of the following is not part of CHAP's process of accreditation and certification?

(A) Visit to the site

(B) Review by a board

(C) Recommendation by a nurse executive

(D) Correction plan

(135) What is the organization charged with reviewing and evaluating HMOs based on employers' data?

(A) US Bureau of Census

(B) US Bureau of Labor and Statistics

(C) National Committee for Quality Assurance

(D) US Agency for Health-Care Research and Quality

(136) Which nurse demonstrated the effectiveness of relationship skills when she secured supplies and other help for those injured in the Crimean War?

(A) Elizabeth Blackwell

(B) Mildred Montag

(C) Florence Nightingale

(D) Sojourner Truth

(137) Which nurse worked toward alleviating incompetence and obtained help for soldiers injured during the Civil War?

(A) Hannah Ropes

(B) Florence Harding

(C) Mary Adelaide

(D) Hildegard Peplau

(138) Who was the individual responsible for forming the first nurses' organization in the United States?

(A) Florence Nightingale

(B) Dr. Joseph DeeLee

(C) Mary Seacole

(D) Isabel Hampton

(139) Which document provides the legal definition of nursing and sets out the profession's scope?

(A) US labor laws

(B) The Emergency Medical and Treatment Labor Act

(C) The Nurse Practice Act

(D) The Hill-Burton Act

(140) Who introduced the environmental theory in nursing?

(A) UNEP

(B) Wangari Maathai

(C) Florence Nightingale

(D) Al Gore

(141) Who designed the Nursing Need Theory?

(A) Faye Glenn Abdellah

(B) Virginia Henderson

(C) Lydia Hall

(D) Florence Nightingale

(142) What is the fourth fundamental pattern of knowledge, in addition to empirical, creative, and ethical, according to Barbara Carper?

(A) Scientific

(B) Personal

(C) Esthetic

(D) Spiritual

(143) Which of the following is not an interest link within the nursing paradigm?

(A) The person

(B) The profession

(C) The environment

(D) Religion

(144) Which of the following is true of the health metaparadigm?

(A) It focuses on the health of the patient's family members.

(B) It focuses on the health of the work environment.

(C) It focuses on the patient's wellness and quality of life.

(D) It focuses on staff wellness and quality of life.

(145) What is the meaning of a conceptual framework in nursing?

(A) All the ideas the nursing profession has built over time

(B) The foundational structure of a hospital

(C) The concepts nurse executives learn during training

(D) The structure within which the nursing concepts are linked

(146) What is formed when a theory is symbolically represented through the use of explanations, diagrams, and notations?

(A) A social interaction model

(B) A conceptual model

(C) Information processing model

(D) Computational model

(147) Who is considered a pioneer nurse theorist?

(A) Dr. Christiaan Barnard

(B) Mary Breckinridge

(C) Florence Nightingale

(D) Johann F. Horner

(148) Which of the following is not one of Myra Levine's principles of conservation?

(A) Structural integrity

(B) Personal liberty

(C) Social stability

(D) Personal integrity

(149) Which of the following is not one of Jean Watson's carative factors?

(A) Promotion of teaching-learning

(B) Development of a help-trust relationship

(C) Promotion of feelings expression

(D) Promotion of economic-health welfare

(150) Who created the Science of Unitary Human Beings theory?

(A) Florence Nightingale

(B) Martha Rogers

(C) Edith Cavell

(D) Sarah E. Edmonds

Test 2: Answers and Explanations

(1) (D) The mix of skills among the nursing staff

There are different categories of personnel in nursing, and the proportion of each type as a percentage of the entire staff at the institution reflects on the capacity of the institution to provide quality services.

(2) (D) The individual should receive mentorship and support.

During peer review, it is not enough to establish if a staff member provided a service differently from the standards expected. It is also important to establish if the variation had any adverse consequences on a patient.

(3) (D) Learning-related and survival-related anxiety

During this stage, people feel dissatisfied and start to question their beliefs. Soon, anxiety caused by the struggle to survive develops. When a patient is required to learn new strategies, this may also lead to learning-related anxiety.

(4) (C) Analyzing vulnerability to hazards

This analysis seeks to identify any potential danger that could disrupt health-care services if an emergency arises. It helps prepare for eventualities like a fire outbreak, plane crash, terrorist attack, and other such threats.

(5) (B) Analyze this rate based on the class the job falls under

The analysis would show the departments or units with low, medium, or high staff turnover. The department with the highest turnover would be addressed, starting with seeking the reason through surveys and/or interviews. After that, new methods of staff retention could be discussed.

(6) (B) Cross-training staff

The cross-training ensures that whichever unit has a staff shortage can be assisted by staff from the other department. It is also encouraged that staff from different units train alongside one another because it helps enhance staff relationships. They also become familiar with equipment and medications, as well as treatments used in the different units.

(7) (C) Acknowledging the important role that patients play

The stages a health-care provider undertakes to engage a patient include believing that the role of the patient is important; possessing the capacity to do something about the patient's needs; doing something to improve the patient's health; and finally, forging ahead even when under stress.

(8) (C) You should treat people the way they prefer to be treated.

The rule is about focusing on the betterment of others as opposed to yourself. You need to respect others, take time to find out what their needs are, and take their views or responses into consideration.

(9) (B) 30 percent

The affected employer is not obliged to officially recognize the existence of the union at that juncture. If the employer does not show recognition for the union, the next step is an appeal to the National Labor Relations Board by the union to have the signatures verified and an election date set.

(10) (A) Restraining and driving

Forces credited with driving change include leaders, competition, and incentives. Forces that restrain change include negative attitudes, inadequate funds, under-equipped facilities, and outright hostility. If the two forces are in balance, then matters are in equilibrium.

(11) (D) Focusing on enhancing relations with others

When using this approach, you try to get people to cooperate and do what others, normally the majority, want. In a power-coercive approach, authoritarian methods are used to impose change. The other major approach is known as rational-empirical. It uses data to provide information meant to influence people into accepting the proposed change.

(12) (A) Problems of a specific nature

PDSA is not applied to problems that cut across an entire organization. Its simplicity fits problems that are specific. It involves three stages: Plan (problem identification) – setting goals, brainstorming and collecting data; Do – generating solutions and identifying one for trial; and Act – identifying required changes, adopting them, and continuously monitoring.

(13) (C) Estimating practitioner supply in the health-care sector

The basis is the training enrollment number and the number of those who graduate at the end of the course. Nurse executives usually find this estimation method helpful as they survey local training institutions because they can predict whether or not their institutions are likely to face a workforce shortage in the near future.

(14) (C) Conduct verifications from the primary sources

This entails acquiring employee transcripts and contacting agencies charged with issuing certifications directly. Copies of valid licenses and other credentials also need to be sourced, and contact must be made with previous employers. In some institutions, this process of verifying the credentials of newly hired employees is contracted to an organization that specializes in this type of work.

(15) (C) Education, performance ability, competence, and licensure

Licensure must be current per the relevant board. Education is in reference to education and residencies, as well as internships and fellowships, and all other forms of professional knowledge and skills acquired professionally. Competence is given by one's peers, while performance ability refers to how well one demonstrates the capacity to carry out duties per his/her credentials.

(16) (D) Provide guidelines and training

Staff members need guidelines and worksheets to use in organizing information. SBAR is an acronym for Situation Background Assessment Recommendations. *Situation* involves name and age, MD, and diagnosis. *Background* involves medical history, ongoing therapy, and such. *Assessment* involves systems review, and completed and required tasks. *Recommendations* are made for a health-care plan review, precautions, etc.

(17) (C) Performance, outcome, structure/technology, and patient experience

The measures are *performance*, whose basis is the set of practices meant to enhance health-care outcomes; *outcome*, whose basis is the achievement of positive results; *patient experience*, whose basis is how satisfied patients feel after receiving care; and *structures or technology*, whose basis is the health-care facilities plus equipment used by health-care providers.

(18) (D) Altered behavior

Four elements comprise the cycle of the theory: input, throughput or processes, output, and feedback. Anything fed into the system, like knowledge, is input. Actions taken in transforming input, like one's experiences, are processes or throughput. What comes out after input processing is output. Feedback, such as praise or support, is information usable in system evaluation.

(19) (C) Coercive power

If a nurse executive uses coercive power, nurses believe he/she does not respect their views or ideas and assume the nurse executive's reaction toward their dissent would most likely be unpleasant. Such staff members may remain silent but end up not cooperating.

(20) (D) Requesting a proposal

Once a proposal request is issued, feedback is usually as varied as the vendors are, with equipment, services, and costs varying. On the contrary, when a quotation request is issued in relation to products or services required, factors like the equipment will be similar to all the vendors, with the cost meant to serve as the determining factor.

(21) (B) Determine tasks that non-RNs can handle

Non-RNs can perform tasks such as transportation, providing personal hygiene services and related care to patients, searching for required equipment, taking patients' routine vitals, and taking patients' specimens to the laboratory.

(22) (C) Console and support the nurse

This culture acknowledges there are differences among three kinds of errors. When it comes to human error, staff may have made a mistake inadvertently, and retraining and other support may help. The second error involves taking unwarranted risks, and coaching and discouraging such risk-taking could help. Reckless error is deliberate, so punitive action may be taken.

(23) (B) Measure outcomes

These are the outcomes that indicate whether implemented changes have had any impact on the provision of health-care services. This includes reimbursement and reporting, complications rate, hospital-stay durations, rehospitalization rate, and health-care costs.

(24) (A) Provide ladders for career growth

Staff should be informed that there is a definite structure that they can advance along within the institution, effectively furthering their careers. Be aware that some strategies, though they increase morale, do not result in greater staff retention. These include providing education-related benefits.

(25) (C) An advanced practice nurse

During the patient's stay at the health institution, the APRN coordinates different health-care providers, including the patient's doctor, therapist, and others. Once that patient has been discharged, the APN serves as the case manager and sees to the patient's continued care while at home.

(26) (C) 30 percent

This percentage is per the Bureau of Labor Statistics, and employers need to take it into account whenever considering the cost of hiring staff. The benefits include medical, vision, and dental insurance; malpractice and disability insurance; workers' compensation; sick days; and vacation time.

(27) (C) 20 months

Annual cost of the employee = $100,000; percentage time = 0.15/15%; efficiency estimate = 0.30/30%. Multiply the numbers to get $4,500. Divide the cost of equipment, $90,000, by $4,500. This gives you 20.

(28) (A) Selling and telling, delegating. and participating

Telling does not motivate staff. Selling is somewhat motivating, as the explanation is given by the leader, who also answers any questions. Participating provides a reasonable level of motivation, as followers participate in discussions on needs and decision-making. Delegating is the most motivating strategy because staff become the decision-makers.

(29) (B) Cost-benefit analysis

This analysis shows the costs involved in the payment of overtime and the financial benefits of hiring additional staff on a full-time basis. The cost-effectiveness analysis is not monetary. Studies of efficacy are meant to identify the best intervention after comparing several cost-benefit analyses. Cost-utility is almost monetarily non-quantifiable.

(30) (D) A needs assessment should be conducted.

This initial step helps establish the most appropriate content. Among the measures to be taken, one should be a staff survey. The coordinator should detail the objectives and techniques to be used in delivery, develop the lesson plans, schedule classes, and make evaluations.

(31) (D) IRF-PAI

The PAI needed is the Inpatient Rehabilitation Facility-Patient Assessment Instrument—IRF-PAI. This document should contain a record of the condition of the patient and the nature of rehabilitative health-care services required.

(32) (B) Statistical discrimination

Statistically, most women's childbearing years are when they are in their mid-twenties. That is why the discrimination by the nurse executive is termed statistical.

(33) (C) Using several methods

Allowing different methods of reporting means whistleblowers can use the method most convenient to them. It also shows that the institution is serious about valuing whistleblowing. State and federal laws pertaining to whistleblowing are not always helpful, as some are contradictory or selective with regards to their application.

(34) (C) 10

The nurse executive's control span is equal to the number of employees who report to him/her directly. That does not alter the fact that everyone else is still the nurse executive's responsibility.

(35) (D) Targeted marketing

Whatever data is available for different demographics can be used to determine the people most likely to benefit from the institution's services. Data on consumers is very helpful in this regard, and when a given population is identified, marketing campaigns can be better targeted.

(36) (B) Create a sense of urgency

Urgency involves encouraging other people to accept the proposed change and emphasizing the importance of altering the state of affairs. A team is then formed to drive the change, set the appropriate vision plus strategy, communicate why the change is valuable, empower people, and remove barriers. The team can then begin to create short-term achievements.

(37) (D) Behaviorally anchored rating scale

BARS has descriptions specific to every point on the scale. For instance, leadership may be assessed on a 1-to-4 scale, where 1 means a total lack of interpersonal skills and 4 means outstanding skills.

(38) (B) 0.5 FTE

0.5 FTE stands for half full-time equivalent, as full time is taken to be 40 hours of work per week in a 52-week-long year, including holidays.

(39) (B) Providing unbiased hiring opportunities so that all qualified candidates are considered

Quota systems are illegal in the United States. Among the best efforts to enhance affirmative action is to increase opportunities for outreach in a bid to enhance staff diversity.

(40) (D) Collaborative bargaining

The bargaining types used in negotiations include distributive, where one side must win and the other lose; integrative, where parties collaborate and everyone leaves the table a winner; and mix, which combines attributes of distributive and integrative bargaining.

(41) (B) Neither the reviewer nor the writer knew the identity of the other.

Not knowing the writer's identity allows for genuine criticism, as opposed to when the reviewer knows the writer's identity and may, therefore, not be as up front with critiques.

(42) (C) Three years

CHNA is expected to be carried out every three years, and the hospital is required to publish the findings on the institution's website. The hospital also must implement processes geared toward meeting the needs identified during the assessment.

(43) (D) Healthgrades

Healthgrades is very helpful to users considering that every month there are around 20 million questions asked by different people. It is also helpful to consumers of health-care services because they can review doctors of all types, including dentists.

(44) (C) Availability of ready information and practice drills

Drills are important because it is easy to forget how to respond to large-scale disasters, since these are not common occurrences. It is recommended that disaster-preparedness drills be carried out at least once every year, with special emphasis on the command chain.

(45) (C) The requirements mandated for reporting and the population of patients

The importance of compliance lies in both the reimbursement and ratings of the health institution, as well as the institution's accreditation. As much as possible, it is preferable that the results identified for data collection be directly linked to the mission of the organization.

(46) (D) Risky

The major question that should be asked pertains to what the worst eventuality might be and how the institution would handle it. These questions help in reviewing every necessary step and identifying existing weaknesses, which then should be addressed as a matter of priority.

(47) (C) Address the worrying behavior and provide resources

It is important that the nurse not be judgmental when attending to patients who want to have their way. Instead, the nurse should provide the patient with facts and then offer any required resources, such as referrals to support groups.

(48) (C) HIE

The Health Information Exchange (HIE) enables information to be communicated securely among health personnel. It also enables health-care providers to request health information pertaining to a given patient or to personally search for it. Also, patients have some level of control over whether or not their information is shared.

(49) (B) Insurance coverage for preexisting health conditions

No patient should be denied insurance because of a preexisting health condition. If already insured, such a person cannot be dropped. Also, parents can cover their dependent children until they are 26 years old. Under this patients' bill of rights, certain preventive care services, like mammograms or physical examinations, are covered.

(50) (C) Nine

Among the nine measures, five of the required are ED-1 and ED-2, VTE-6, IMM-2, and PC-01.

(51) (D) Proximity and research, as well as adverse effects and accuracy

Evidence gathered through research should support the recommended interventions. As for proximity, there should be a close link between the process in use and the outcome. Accuracy means the level of the intervention's effectiveness should be measured with great precision. The measure should avoid any negative effects, including those produced inadvertently.

(52) (A) Encourage others to make decisions

It is important to appreciate that every level of the institution has people with leadership qualities, and these ought to be nurtured. Leadership that is pervasive manifests respect as well as trust in other staff, and it encourages them to be proactive in finding solutions to issues at their own level. It is the opposite of the leader-follower model.

(53) (A) Look for any opportunities to get grants

It is incumbent upon any nurse executive seeking funding to demonstrate how cost-effective a proposed project is expected to be. The board focuses mainly on the cost involved in a proposal, so the accrued benefits should be shown to be worthwhile.

(54) (B) Form a journal club

By joining a journal club, the nurses will get into the habit of reading things like medical articles, and then one of them can report on those articles at group meetings. The entire group can then brainstorm on how that information can be utilized when providing health-care services.

(55) (A) The constructionist principle

The constructionist principle finds a direct correlation between what people do and what their beliefs are, simultaneously addressing the institution being inquired about.

(56) (C) Informed consent is not necessary.

Although there is a need to protect research subjects, the provision is meant to ensure researchers do not face undue pressure. The common-rule revision took effect in 2018.

(57) (B) Priority, performance, and philosophy

Philosophy is about looking at education for patients as a good investment, while priority indicates the importance of patients receiving education, not only for those patients but also for the quality of nursing in general. Performance is necessary for nurses to be knowledgeable and skilled in providing education to the patients.

(58) (B) Mentoring

An individual serving as a mentor is usually qualified in advanced nursing, and other times such an individual has undergone training in evidence-based research. In short, a mentor serves as a great resource for staff.

(59) (A) Resolution of problems

It was Peplau's belief that it is important that there be a good relationship between nurses and the patients they are treating and that the two collaborate.

(60) (C) Gradual testing of changes

This means that the system is tested in sections as opposed to all at once. This is done in a manner that makes it possible to note any weaknesses or problems.

Checking small areas at a time also makes it relatively easy to note those areas where staff need more training.

(61) (C) To modify methods in order to increase the speed of response

The idea is to double or triple the quality-enhancement rate. Rapid action teams are used to find and test solutions rather than engaging in analysis. Teams have meetings for six weeks, with the first week focusing on review of information and clarification of opportunities. The last week involves implementation.

(62) (D) Personal physicians

PCMHs seek to minimize patient complications so that there is minimal need for patients to be hospitalized. Since the teams at PCMHs render different levels of health care, from acute to hospice, costs are greatly reduced.

(63) (C) A nervous state

The act of lip licking is a sign of nervousness, and the person might also be avoiding direct eye contact while staring elsewhere. Hand rubbing is an attempt by the person to comfort himself/herself.

(64) (B) A scattergram

A scattergram has X and Y axes, with X representing age and Y representing admissions. The scattergram demonstrates how admissions are done in various units per the dates and patients' ages. There is a data point for every admission, which corresponds to the age of every patient. Charting the data helps determine if a pattern exists.

(65) (C) Eliminate them

The intention is to simplify processes and maintain their integrity. Some stages can be eliminated when more modern equipment is bought, which allows for a design change. Changes can also be made to the environment, where the process is carried out exactly at the point where care is given as opposed to a different venue.

(66) (B) Establishing rapport

Rapport can be established by asking questions that are not related to work, like inquiring how the person's child is doing. After that light conversation, you can inquire the person's opinion regarding work—the areas that are going well and those that are problematic.

(67) (C) Passive-aggressive style

To identify passive-aggressiveness, listen for sarcasm. People who are passive-aggressive usually behave as if they agree with the speaker, but once left alone, they act in a manner that undermines the other person's authority.

(68) (A) Some of the patients' information on their health is shared by various ACO providers among themselves.

ACO is an acronym for Accountable Care Organization, and sometimes patients are assigned to them via Medicare. When this happens, patients can expect information to be shared among different health-care providers under the ACO. Patients under ACO are not eligible to become participants of the Medicare Advantage plan.

(69) (D) Admitted from a homeless shelter

Homelessness is an indicator, and so are squalid living conditions, surviving on limited income, and depending on other people to provide care. Where violence is concerned, the case is reportable and must be managed in a more comprehensive manner.

(70) (A) Empathy

Empathy is part of a person's emotional intelligence. The other elements are self-awareness, self-regulation, motivation, and social skills.

(71) (C) Reflecting

The aim is to get that staff member to come to terms with his/her fears or concerns. When one reflects, it is an indication of having paid attention, a behavior that ends up encouraging the other person to open up more and air his/her personal views.

(72) (C) Suggest that the evaluations remain anonymous

The reason these evaluations need to remain anonymous is that the people carrying out the evaluations might be afraid of possible repercussions if the individuals whose performance is being reviewed were known to them.

(73) (B) She respects the suggestions given by the speaker.

Although all signs indicate respect for the subordinate, the nurse executive is not obliged to adhere to the suggestions made by that staff member. At the same time, if the nurse executive does not concur with any suggestions given, it is important that she not respond in a negative manner.

(74) (D) Encouraging staff to identify any problems and come up with solutions

The idea is to encourage every team member to participate actively in the change process. In comparison to the empirical-rational model that is based on facts and figures, this participatory model of arriving at rational conclusions or decisions is slower.

(75) (C) It triggers change in other areas.

Change in one place also calls for changes in different areas because different systems of a whole are normally interrelated. The model in question is termed STAR because the diagram resembles a star. Its five points are strategy, structure, human resources, incentives, and information or decision-making.

(76) (B) The reason for the impending changes

Giving a reason is important because staff members have a habit of being more cooperative once they are aware of the reason for the actions they have been asked to take. As a nurse executive, you need to endeavor to show your staff the rationale behind actions you suggest and, where possible, give evidence.

(77) (D) The geographical location of the population that is targeted

The areas where Medicare permits telehealth are classified as Health Professional Shortage Areas, per the country's census bureau. Nevertheless, some programs under Medicare, like Medicare Advantage, support delivery of services via telehealth when it relates to the management of chronic ailments. In the latter case, the patient incurs a greater cost.

(78) (D) The rate of individual health facility utilization in the city

Outcome assessments for large areas, like states or countries, merge data to reflect averages, which means that data on small areas is not accurately reflected in such assessments. A small-area analysis reflects more accurate data on small areas, so it is used for epidemiologic rates and data on hospital utilization.

(79) (B) Throughput

The five elements of a system are input, throughput, output, evaluation, and feedback. According to Bertalanffy, the five elements in the system all interact to achieve various goals. When one element is changed, the rest of the elements are also affected, and outcomes are consequently altered.

(80) (C) 26 workweeks

FMLA grants workers who have spouses, children, or parents in the military a 26 workweek period in a year as a Military Caregiver Leave.

(81) (A) Strategic goals

Lean Six Sigma is a combination of two different continuous improvement methods, Six Sigma and lean. It focuses process improvements on a strategic goal instead of a single project, with its main goal being to minimize waste and errors within an organization.

(82) (D) Costs incurred from products or services used to prevent errors or failures, such as evaluation and monitoring

Conformance costs are related to error prevention, such as evaluation and monitoring costs. Nonconformance costs are costs related to failures, defects, and errors, such as infections, malpractice, lost time, and poor access to services.

(83) (B) Breach

A breach occurs when staff members fail to perform their duties according to acceptable practice standards. Duty refers to the legal obligation or responsibility that one party has to another, while causation is proof that breach of duty caused harm.

(84) (D) Gross negligence

Generally, negligence is said to occur when a caregiver fails to provide services that are in line with the established standards of care. There are various kinds of negligence, including gross negligence, contributory negligence, comparative negligence, and negligent conduct.

(85) (B) Cost-benefit analysis

This type of analysis uses the average cost of the event and cost of interventions to determine savings. Cost-effective analysis determines how effective an invention is, while cost-utility analysis measures benefits to society.

(86) (C) It is a plan that is authorized by Medicare and administered by private insurance firms.

Medicare Advantage is a Medicare-approved plan that is provided by private insurance firms. This managed care plan is required to follow the established rules provided by Medicare, and Medicare pays a fixed monthly amount to the insurance company for the enrolled beneficiaries.

(87) (A) Its vision statement

An organization's vision statement indicates its commitment to strategic planning and includes its future goals.

(88) (C) Congratulating a staff member for demonstrating exemplary skills in nursing that prevented an accident from occurring

Providing a monetary incentive ,such as a salary increase, is one way of showing recognition, but this kind of recognition tends to be automatically triggered. The better way of showing meaningful recognition is recognizing real contributions and providing individual feedback.

(89) (A) Clients' safety

Clients' safety is always the main area of concern in risk management. An effective risk management plan includes goals, program scope, authorities, policies, referrals/data sources, documentation/reporting, program evaluation, activities integration, and charts/diagrams.

(90) (B) OSHA

The Occupational Safety and Health Administration is the governmental agency that determines the Bloodborne Pathogens Standards and other standards in the workplace.

(91) (D) The organization and its processes

The Continuous Quality Improvement model focuses more on the organization, processes, and systems than on any one individual. This model uses the experimental method to improve services while utilizing tools like brainstorming, multi-voting, storyboarding, charts, diagrams, and meetings.

(92) (C) Within 27 days

The Inpatient Rehabilitation Facility Patient Assessment Instrument on Medicare Part C (Medicare Advantage) or Medicare Part A fee-for-service should be sent to the CMS National Assessment Collection Database within 27 days.

(93) (B) During the American Revolution

The motivation behind opening the dispensary was that the army was losing more men from illness than from being shot. A good example is smallpox, which normally kills a third of those infected. But with soldiers being inoculated, chances of survival rose significantly.

(94) (B) Clara Barton and Sojourner Truth

Barton and Truth were both nurses and activists. The public appreciated their role in tending to soldiers during the American Civil War, alongside others like Harriet Tubman.

(95) (D) During the Spanish-American War

During the Spanish-American War, there were already schools of nursing in existence, but Isabel Robb designed a plan geared toward the management of nurses for better service delivery.

(96) (B) They had to be well-behaved and not married.

Nurses trained at the army nursing school that was established by the US government in 1918 were expected to be well-behaved and single. The training was recommended as a substitute for the utilization of nurse aides at army hospitals.

(97) (A) It was responsible for the creation of the Nurse Cadet Corps in the United States.

In addition to introducing the country's US Nurse Cadet Corps, the Bolton Act also allocated funds amounting to a $160 million dollars for use by 1,125 schools of nursing, which included those that trained African Americans.

(98) (A) Triaging the injured soldiers at every treatment stage

The nurses focused their care on soldiers, ensuring proper triage. This meant the nurses performed resuscitation in a timely manner and prioritized the rest of the care for the injured as required.

(99) (A) ICN

ICN stands for International Council of Nurses, which works toward enhancing the welfare of individual nurses, organizations for nurses, and their governing institutions. It addresses both the social and economic aspects of welfare.

(100) (C) The American Nurses Association

The ANA is a professional body whose role involves the advancement and protection of nursing as a profession. The organization was established in 1896, but at the time it was referred to as the Nurses Associated Alumnae.

(101) (B) The American Association of Colleges of Nursing

The AACN is the body through which issues pertaining to nurse education in the United States are channeled. Not only does the organization set the required standards for all nurses, but it also monitors training schools to ensure they are imparting the right skills to meet the standards.

(102) (A) The Commission on Collegiate Nursing Education

The CCNE was established to accord accreditation to nurse graduates and those in residency. The country's education secretary recognizes the CCNE as the agency in charge of such accreditation nationally.

(103) (B) The National Council of State Boards of Nursing

The NCSBN is the nonprofit body through which all the country's organizations dealing with issues of nursing collaborate for the enhancement of health-care provision, health, and public safety.

(104) (C) Sigma Theta Tau International

The STTI was established in 1922 at Indiana University by a group of six nursing students. The number of those inducted has since exceeded 250,000, membership being solely through invitation. One hundred and twenty thousand of these members are active, with over 7,000 of them holding PhDs or master's degrees.

(105) (C) Putting pressure on employers to pay high salaries to nurses

The NSNA focuses on the welfare of nursing students as they prepare for licensure and advance in their education and training, but it does not concern itself with matters of remuneration.

(106) (D) Mentoring students in high school who would like to acquire a nursing associate degree later

The NOADN does not go to schools to mentor potential nurses. It addresses the quality of education provided by associate degree programs and the quality of service provided by nurses with associate degrees once in the field.

(107) (A) AHA

The American Organization of Nurse Executives (AONE) falls under the American Hospitals Association (AHA) as a subsidiary. The AONE is responsible for the design and management of health-care services provided by nurses across the country.

(108) (B) NANDA-International

NANDA is the acronym for North American Nursing Diagnosis Association, whose name has been adjusted to NANDA-International. This organization, which was established in 1982, is in charge of standardizing terminologies used in the field of nursing.

(109) (D) Preventative services

Preventative services in the health-care sector are low in cost, and sometimes they are provided free of charge.

(110) (C) Age of the patient

The age of the patient is not a factor when health-care providers are considering rationing of health care, but the other three options are important factors to be considered.

(111) (A) It releases funds in advance when there is an insured patient in need of health-care services.

Health-care services must be provided by a physician or other providers who have a contract with the HMO before funds can be released.

(112) (C) The nurse providing community-based care needs to be a relative of the patient.

Option (C) is not true. The important thing is that the nurse does the utmost to understand the patient and the values of the family and community.

(113) (C) The amount managed care pays for a patient depends on what other plans pay for similar services.

Option (C) is not true because the amount the managed care plan pays is dependent on the rules set by its network of health-care providers.

(114) (B) Under capitation, the PCP is paid by the state government.

Option (B) is untrue because the primary care provider (PCP) receives payment from the insurer or physicians' association.

(115) (C) It is designed to monitor the patient's kidney function.

The wearable monitor, which is also implantable, is meant to provide a reading of the patient's physiological parameters. From them, the doctor can determine if the patient's condition is improving or deteriorating. The monitor does not assess kidney function.

(116) (B) Arm

The arm is one of the locations recommended for injecting insulin. The other options—insulin vial, insulin pen, and insulin pump—are methods by which insulin is administered beneath the skin.

(117) (C) Nursery

Primary health-care organizations, like community hospitals and nurse practitioners' clinics, provide essential health care. They are the first place patients normally visit with medical concerns. Institutions are termed secondary when they can handle illnesses of a more complex nature, like pneumonia or a broken bone. They are tertiary when their care is specialized, like having an ICU or a trauma unit.

(118) (B) A ward that admits patients for a short period; sometimes for just 48 hours

SSU stands for short-stay unit. These units take patients who are intended to be hospitalized for a short period, ordinarily for fewer than two days.

(119) (D) It is not licensed to handle obstetric cases.

Acute-care hospitals are licensed to diagnose and treat obstetric cases.

(120) (B) It is limited to providing medicines and any necessary injections.

Long-term care involves taking care of the patient's medical and nonmedical needs, including physical therapy, counseling, and others. Some of the services under long-term care, such as the modification of a patient's home to accommodate a disability, are not covered by Medicare, but there is insurance for long-term care.

(121) (B) The intensity of care a patient requires

Some hospitals determine the number of staff to put on duty depending on the patients' acuity in a unit, meaning depending on the degree of care the patients require.

(122)(B) Patients who need it are never hospitalized.

Option (B) is untrue because patients requiring subacute care can be treated as either outpatients or inpatients.

(123)(C) Skilled nursing care

Skilled nursing care has to be given by a qualified and duly licensed health professional like an RN. For Medicare or Medicaid to pay for services, they must have been recommended by a physician.

(124)(B) Bathing and selecting suitable clothes to wear for the day

ADL stands for Activities of Daily Living, the basic things that a person normally does without much effort and without the need for help. These include eating and bathing. dressing, toileting, transferring (the capacity to walk), and continence.

(125) (B) Taking the patient to visit as many friends as possible before dying

The care services offered in a hospice include those of a medical, social, and spiritual nature. The patients and their relatives receive nursing services and spiritual support.

(126) (C) To help patients regain their health and function as normally as possible

Rehab services are meant to rehabilitate the patient so that he/she can regain functionality that deteriorated during illness or injury.

(127) (B) When patients are receiving ambulatory care

Ambulatory care is the same as outpatient care, meaning the patient is treated at a clinic or hospital and goes home the same day. Ambulatory care patients are not hospitalized.

(128) (D) Nurses cannot provide intravenous services to patients under home health care.

Option (D) is not true. All forms of treatments can be provided to patients under home health care, as long as a doctor has recommended them. The services could be administration of medicine, dressing of wounds, IV-based therapy, physical or speech therapy, and others.

(129) (B) Community hospitals are run by the federal government.

Community hospitals are variously owned, the greatest proportion—around 58 percent—being run on a nonprofit basis. The remaining proportion is divided between those run as profit-earning organizations and those owned and run by the government. Community hospitals are sometimes referred to as general hospitals.

(130) (B) Immunology center

Immunology services can be safely offered at any level of health-care provision, including the primary level. The other three options are found in tertiary care hospitals because they require specialized care and equipment.

(131) (D) They specialize in providing specific types of health care.

One specialty hospital can specialize in carrying out orthopedic surgeries, another can specialize in ophthalmology, another in obstetrics, and so on.

(132) (D) It is in charge of regulating health-care insurance coverage.

Provision of insurance services is regulated through guidelines issued by the National Association of Insurance Commissioners and then adopted by states to become legal.

(133) (A) It is the sole body charged with accreditation of health-care institutions.

JCAHO stands for the Joint Commission on Accreditation of Healthcare Organizations. Although it is the leading accreditation body in the United States, it is not the only one. Others include the Accreditation Commission for Health Care and the Community Health Accreditation Program.

(134) (C) Recommendation by a nurse executive

Other elements of the process of accreditation and certification by CHAP include application, readiness for a visit to the site, contract signing, and actual certification.

(135) (C) National Committee for Quality Assurance

The National Committee for Quality Assurance reviews HMOs on the basis of the Healthcare Effectiveness Data and Information Set (HEDIS).

(136) (C) Florence Nightingale

During the Crimean War, Florence Nightingale used her relationship skills by engaging the powerful people she knew in government to secure not only supplies but also personnel to help the injured.

(137) (A) Hannah Ropes

During the Civil War, Hannah Ropes contacted some influential individuals in Washington, and as a result, she raised the standard of care wounded soldiers were receiving. At the time, she was head matron at Washington's Union Hotel Hospital.

(138) (D) Isabel Hampton

Isabel Hampton helped form the ANA, a successor to the Nurses Associated Alumnae of the United States and Canada, an organization she headed as president since its formation in 1896.

(139)(C) The Nurse Practice Act

In addition to providing a definition of nursing and indicating its scope, the Nurse Practice Act also sets out the authority and power of nursing boards.

(140)(C) Florence Nightingale

The environmental theory in nursing posits that patients' environments can be adjusted in a manner that is supportive of each individual's personal recovery.

(141) (B) Virginia Henderson

The Nursing Need Theory designed by Virginia Henderson focuses on the need for nurses to help patients meet their basic needs and to be creative when implementing doctors' plan of care so that the needs specific to an individual patient can be adequately met.

(142)(B) Personal

Scientific knowledge is the same as empirical knowledge, and an aesthetic pattern is the same as a creative one. There is no spiritual knowledge pattern among those identified by Barbara Carper.

(143)(D) Religion

There are normally four such interest links in the nursing paradigm: the person, the profession, health, and the environment.

(144) (C) It focuses on the patient's wellness and quality of life.

In addition to focusing on the patient's wellness and quality of life, the metaparadigm of health also addresses the accessibility of health-care services to the patient.

(145) (D) The structure within which the nursing concepts are linked

The important concepts of the person, the environment, health and the nursing profession are linked in the nursing framework.

(146) (B) A conceptual model

Researchers often use conceptual models in nursing to design and conduct their investigations. A conceptual model can correctly be viewed as a theoretical model that gives coherence to the way events and processes relate.

(147) (C) Florence Nightingale

Florence Nightingale is considered the pioneer nurse theorist. She is recognized for the way she described nursing as being an art as well as a science.

(148) (B) Personal liberty

Myra Levine is another nurse theorist, and her fourth principle is energy conservation.

(149)(D) Promotion of economic-health welfare

Jean Watson's other carative factors include humanistic-altruistic systems of value, decision-making by solving problems, promotion of a supportive environment, and helping with the human need for gratification.

(150)(B) Martha Rogers

Martha Rogers developed a theory that views the person as a unit that is fully integrated so that its value surpasses that of its constituent parts in total.

Test 3: Questions

(1) Which act helps ensure that an organization with a workforce of 50 employees will provide unpaid leave to employees without risking their jobs?

(A) The National Labor Relations Act

(B) The Americans with Disabilities Act

(C) The Fair Labor Standards Act

(D) The Family and Medical Leave Act

(2) An employee has to take leave to care for his infant. According to the Family and Medical Leave Act, how many weeks can the employee take an unpaid absence without risking his position at the organization?

(A) Twelve weeks

(B) Three weeks

(C) Eight weeks

(D) Two weeks

(3) According to the Family and Medical Leave Act, what is the special concession if an employee applies to take care of a spouse who is a service member?

(A) Additional benefits and responsibilities

(B) A new position with a salary and benefits commensurate with the previous job

(C) Concurrent benefits extended to 26 weeks per year

(D) No special concessions

(4) The Americans with Disabilities Act is intended to ensure that ________.

(A) The civil rights of Americans with any kind of mental disability are respected and those individuals are given an equal chance of employment

(B) The social rights of less privileged people are protected

(C) Civil rights of any American with a sound mind are respected

(D) No equal opportunities are granted to Americans with any kind of mental disability

(5) What is the role of nurse executives when it comes to carrying out the stipulations of the Americans with Disabilities Act?

(A) They should ensure modes of communication are convenient for disabled people, such as providing devices for helping people with hearing and vision problems.

(B) They should make sure that ADA stipulations are adhered to and, if they are not, make the necessary recommendations.

(C) They should provide transport services that include wheelchairs for people with disabilities.

(D) They should help install elevators and ramps.

(6) How is the overtime rate calculated according to the Fair Labor Standard Act (FLSA)?

(A) A minimum hourly rate of $2.13 should be given for overtime.

(B) Overtime begins counting after 50 working hours every week. The calculations are done at one and a half times the standard rate.

(C) The rates for overtime remain the same as the standard rate.

(D) Overtime begins counting after 40 working hours every week. Calculations are done at one and a half times the standard rate.

(7) How does the state minimum wage differ from the federal minimum wage according to the FLSA?

(A) Hospitals have no partial exemptions regarding overtime and no authority to pay below minimum wage.

(B) The state minimum wage is always $2.13 above the federal minimum wage.

(C) The state can have its minimum wage above the federal minimum. Employees are entitled to higher salaries if state and federal wage laws vary.

(D) The state and federal minimum wage have no difference.

(8) What minimum wage should employees be paid under the McNamara-O'Hara Service Contract Act?

(A) Any contractor handling a contract worth more than $2,500 should pay the minimum wage according to that time.

(B) Employees should be paid the minimum or better wage if the contract's worth is below $2,500.

(C) Any contractor handling a federal contract worth over $100,000 must pay overtime at one and a half times per hour.

(D) Employees should be paid the minimum wage if the contract's worth exceeds $2,500.

(9) What act is responsible for ensuring that employers do not discriminate against employees based on their gender, race, country of origin, religion or pregnancy?

(A) The Equal Employment Opportunity Commission

(B) The Federal Wage Garnishment Law

(C) The 1964 Civil Rights Act, Title VII

(D) The 1991 Civil Rights Act

(10) An employee is above age 40. Which of the following laws protects her rights?

(A) The 1967 ADEA

(B) The 1972 Rehabilitation Act

(C) The 1991 Civil Rights Act

(D) The 2008 GINA

(11) What is your role as a nurse executive when it comes to applying OSHA policies?

(A) Oversee the policies for infection control

(B) Comply with state regulations, even if they're more stringent than the ones set by OSHA

(C) Ensure devices intended for medical use are safe

(D) Cater to situations where the patients may be exposed to infection

(12) Which of the following is not a form of workers' compensation that benefits employees injured while on duty?

(A) Reimbursement of any cost inflicted during treatment for the injury

(B) Cash as a substitute for wages not earned during the injury or illness

(C) Increase in wages and promotion after the employee rejoins the organization

(D) Benefits paid to next of kin in case the injured employee dies

(13) The Omnibus Budget Reconciliation Act encompasses the Nursing Home Reform Amendments. According to the amendments, patients must be taken care of on a 24-hour basis.

What is the minimum time for RNs on duty in a single day?

(A) Double shift

(B) Half shift

(C) Single shift

(D) No minimum time required

(14) According to the EMTALA, when is the transfer of patients from the ER possible within the hospital or to a different hospital?

(A) The transfer can be made if patients are in an unstable condition and the hospital does not have the resources to take care of them.

(B) The transfer is possible only when patients have been stabilized. If a patient is in labor, the transfer is only allowed when she has delivered both the baby and the placenta.

(C) The transfer can be made if anyone related to the patient demands it.

(D) The transfer can only be made if patients have insurance or can pay their medical bills.

(15) What matters are addressed through the collective bargaining agreement between employees and employers?

(A) Matters revolving around wages and workplace conditions

(B) Timely revisions of the agreements

(C) Discussion on the administrative positions nurse executives hold

(D) The regulations and contracts pertaining to the agreements

(16) Which of the following bargaining types is not a major way of carrying out labor negotiations?

(A) Integrative negotiation

(B) Distributive negotiation

(C) Mixed negotiation

(D) Composite negotiation

(17) Which bargaining type focuses on negotiations in a collaborative environment that help resolve any dispute and help both parties reach a mutual and satisfactory decision?

(A) Composite bargaining

(B) Distributive bargaining

(C) Mixed bargaining

(D) Integrative bargaining

(18) What is your role as a nurse executive during contract negotiations?

(A) Ensure only one party makes the opening statement and the other presents a counterargument.

(B) Ensure that the negotiations are factual and not emotional.

(C) Ensure that the parties state the position they consider to be the most reasonable for the other party.

(D) Ensure there is no room to maneuver during the negotiations.

(19) How is the cost split between both parties when a grievance is presented for arbitration?

(A) The employer or the authoritative entity covers the cost of arbitration.

(B) The immediate supervisor covers the cost of arbitration and neither party pays anything.

(C) The cost of arbitration is split between both parties.

(D) The cost of arbitration is split between the immediate supervisor and both parties.

(20) How many board judges work with the NLRB to help with labor-related cases?

(A) Twenty-eight

(B) Forty

(C) Thirty-two

(D) Twenty

(21) Active listening is a principle of communication. Which of the following statements communicates you are truly empathetic to the other person's situation?

(A) "Maybe this is a blessing in disguise."

(B) "I'm sorry you feel that way."

(C) "I was saddened to hear of your loss. My staff and I send our condolences."

(D) "Try to pull yourself together."

(22) How is two-way communication described between a senior and a junior employee in a hospital?

(A) Progressive

(B) Horizontal

(C) Upward

(D) Vertical

(23) In the sender-receiver feedback loop, why is giving feedback important for communication during the decoding step?

(A) It is the only way the encoder will know that the transmitted message has been received with its intended meaning.

(B) It shows the encoder compiled the message correctly.

(C) The context and interference can only be understood when feedback is given.

(D) It shows the message sent reached the intended recipient.

(24) During an interview for staff hiring, which of the following questions should not be asked?

(A) "How many years of experience do you have?"

(B) "What is your ethnicity?"

(C) "What value can you add to the job position?"

(D) "What soft skills do you think can help you with your position?"

(25) Read the following statement and classify its communication style.

I feel as though your interruption during the staff meeting undermined my authority.

(A) Persuasive

(B) Passive

(C) Assertive

(D) Aggressive

(26) What does a person with a passive communication style avoid in the short term?

(A) Growth opportunities

(B) Conflict

(C) Reaching a mutual decision

(D) Making no statement

(27) It is important to ensure that training provides the staff with diverse skills and that they can test those skills in their time at the health care institution.

What is this type of training called?

(A) Compliance training

(B) Cross-training

(C) Onboarding training

(D) Orientation training

(28) With what does the accordion schedule help nurse executives?

(A) It sets fixed schedules for staff members.

(B) It defines the number of hours and days staff members work.

(C) It ensures that all staff positions are filled daily, even if someone is on leave.

(D) It oversees staff members who break their day into multiple shifts.

(29) Which of the following factors should not be taken into account for the rubrics that indicate a salary range that can help determine the best package for every applicant?

(A) Age of the applicant

(B) Years of experience

(C) Education credits

(D) Special skills

(30) At the development of a plan of performance stage in employee performance management, what must the administration agree on with the employees?

(A) Three to five goals expected by the end of a given period and a success measuring rate

(B) Helping employees train to meet established goals through positive or negative feedback

(C) Assessing individual or group performances annually at the minimum

(D) Agreeing on focusing on matters of priority, providing constructive criticism and using appropriate behavior

(31) A hospital has poor labeling equipment. An employee using the equipment has been showing a downward trend in performance.

What is the main feature of a just culture in employee engagement strategies that can help fix this issue?

(A) Showing employees some consideration and seeing them as humans who can make mistakes.

(B) Giving appropriate coaching to employees who tend to take unwarranted risks.

(C) Focusing on streamlining the system instead of changing employees' behavior.

(D) Taking remedial action or punitive measures.

(32) Which of the following is not a matter crucial to the need for transparency in the workplace?

(A) Disclosure of information

(B) Clarity in disseminating information

(C) Productive meetings between the employee and employer

(D) Communication of information with accuracy

(33) According to the command chain hierarchy, nurse executives come immediately below _________.

(A) The institution governing body

(B) Staff leaders

(C) Senior managers

(D) The chief executive officer

(34) Organizational charts have three formats. Which of the following is not one of those formats?

(A) Matrix format

(B) Hierarchical format

(C) Bottom-up

(D) Flat format

(35) Control span is the number of people that need to be supervised. A narrow control span is defined through the work being performed that _________.

(A) Is mainly of a routine nature

(B) Does not need much direction

(C) Has complex tasks and varies in nature

(D) Has no rules or regulations

(36) As a manager or someone with authority, you will be expected to determine the best control span for your organization.

Which of the following elements helps to determine the best control span?

(A) Organization's size, age of employees, nature of employees' skills, culture in the organization built over time and responsibilities of different supervisors

(B) Organization's size, nature of skills of employees, culture in the organization built over time, the nature of training supervisors have received and the responsibilities of different supervisors

(C) Organization's size, nature of skills of employees, culture in the organization built over time, the nature of training employees have received and the responsibilities of different employees

(D) Organization's size, nature of skills of employees, culture in the organization built over time and the nature of training supervisors have received

(37) What is the major difference between a policy and a procedure?

(A) Procedures explain the "why" of something, whereas policies talk about the "how" of something.

(B) Policies are not flexible, while procedures can be changed.

(C) Policies are clear and concise, but procedures aren't.

(D) Policies have a simple language, whereas procedures have complex language.

(38) What are the four elements of team performance management?

(A) Purpose, outcomes, accountability and outcome management

(B) Reviews, planning, feedback and accountability

(C) Monitoring, communication, collaboration and negotiation

(D) Negotiation, communication, collaboration and conflict management

(39) Which of the following statements is true?

(A) A group cannot be formed to provide therapy or personal support.

(B) Heterogeneous groups comprise members with something in common while having different aspects like gender or age.

(C) Groups of form are homogenous in nature and have specific members that are only part of those groups.

(D) A closed group never welcomes new members but can have changes in group leadership.

(40) Which of the following is not part of the steps that help individuals execute change effectively?

(A) Awareness

(B) Desire

(C) Emotions

(D) Ability

(41) What is an important factor for any people in charge of change management?

(A) They should be objective toward the change and show no personal attachment to whether or not it happens.

(B) They should be concerned about how the change could alter things.

(C) They should have the relevant knowledge and skills to carry out the tasks to bring about the change.

(D) They should allow other individuals to do as they desire.

(42) Nurse executives need to have a good understanding of which of the following factors to bring about effective change management?

(A) How to bring about awareness regarding change management

(B) Their desire to bring about change

(C) ADKAR

(D) The six distinct phases that planned change undergoes

(43) The culture of safety includes all of the following except _____.

(A) Change management

(B) Accountability

(C) Safety gear for ensuring employee safety

(D) Risk management

(44) Which of the following is false regarding risks?

(A) Risks can be avoided

(B) Risks can be monitored

(C) Risks can be desired

(D) Risks can be mitigated

(45) According to the ANA, which of the following is not a part of effective leadership?

(A) Promoting a culture of safety

(B) The satisfaction rate of patients and staff with administration

(C) Being well-versed in federal and state laws

(D) Empowering those who are working under you

(46) Which of the following ensures a safe working environment?

(A) An institution that employs inexperienced staff

(B) An institution that does not believe in training its staff

(C) An institution with policies in place to prevent bullying and other forms of violence

(D) None of the above

(47) Staff empowerment requires good leadership to _______.

(A) Nullify policies that promote punctuality

(B) Provide equal pay without discrimination

(C) Not discriminate based on age or gender

(D) Allow employees a certain level of autonomy per their respective positions

(48) Which of the following ensures staff satisfaction?

(A) Flexible work schedule

(B) Fair wages

(C) Discrimination based on race and religion

(D) Exemption from training and awareness seminars

(49) What continuous process improvement is also known as the Deming Cycle?

(A) The Plan-Do-Check-Act Cycle

(B) Lean Six Sigma

(C) Root cause analysis

(D) Change management

(50) _______________ is a method of process improvement which is used in manufacturing environments.

(A) Lean Six Sigma

(B) The PDCA Cycle

(C) Change management

(D) A root cause analysis

(51) Continuous process improvement and research and practice methods are both part of ________.

(A) Risk management

(B) Change management

(C) Knowledge management

(D) Safety culture

(52) Which continuous process improvement method is considered a preventative measure?

(A) Lean Six Sigma

(B) The PDCA Cycle

(C) Change management

(D) Root cause analysis

(53) How can nurse executives protect the people who serve as subjects in research projects?

(A) They should be able to conduct reviews of relevant literature.

(B) They should be conversant with the laws put in place by the Institutional Review Board (IRB) and FDA.

(C) They should be able to conduct case-controlled studies.

(D) They should know about PICOT, which guides how quantitative questions are designed in any research.

(54) Nurse executives are required to have a strong grasp of the different elements of research in order to be skilled in ________.

(A) Research-subject protection

(B) Research practice and techniques

(C) Change management

(D) Performance enhancement

(55) Which of the following does not qualify as a method through which nurse executives can advocate for the people carrying out research in their institution?

(A) Creating a journal club

(B) Forming an interdisciplinary council that promotes and supports research

(C) Protecting research subjects

(D) Being knowledgeable about writing grants to secure resources to help improve the research being conducted

(56) How can innovations contribute to knowledge management?

(A) They can help implement modern technologies and techniques.

(B) They can help monitor and control risks.

(C) They can help manage changes.

(D) They can help conduct high-quality research.

(57) Why does a nurse executive need to know systems theory?

(A) To ensure performance enhancement

(B) To implement change management

(C) To ensure patients' health and safety

(D) To understand risk management

(58) ____________ is a systems theory that compares organic systems to mechanical systems.

(A) Complex adaptive theory

(B) Innovation management theory

(C) Contingency theory

(D) Bertalanffy's systems theory

(59) Systems whose conditions are subject to change are considered _______.

(A) Unstable

(B) Mechanic

(C) Organic

(D) None of the above

(60) What is not one of the five distinct disciplines of a learning institution?

(A) Shared vision

(B) Team learning

(C) Innovations

(D) Mental models

(61) _________________ is a discipline of a learning organization where an institution is viewed holistically.

(A) Shared vision

(B) Systems thinking

(C) Personal mastery

(D) Mental model

(62) According to CQI, who are internal customers?

(A) The patients

(B) The vendors

(C) The staff

(D) The administrators

(63) _____________ is a performance enhancement model applied to facilitate change in an institution.

(A) FOCUS

(B) TQM

(C) CQI

(D) None of the above.

(64) The ____________ in FOCUS refers to the step where team members brainstorm to resolve problems.

(A) Find

(B) Clarify

(C) Organize

(D) Start

(65) Which of the following is not a clinical outcome?

(A) Patient satisfaction

(B) Employee empowerment

(C) Implementation of safety standards

(D) Compliance with the objectives and goals of the institution

(66) Financial planning usually covers a period of ______.

(A) A decade

(B) Five years

(C) A year

(D) A month

(67) __________ is one of the best ways to ensure financial planning is being implemented.

(A) Expenditure control

(B) Budget management

(C) Evaluation of costs incurred

(D) Enabling feedback on financial performance

(68) Which of the following is not a part of the revenue cycle?

(A) Coding

(B) Collection

(C) Chargemaster

(D) Payer system

(69) ____________ requires a nurse executive to be well-versed in both verbal and nonverbal interactions.

(A) Networking

(B) Effective communication

(C) Financial planning

(D) Making an environment conducive to employee interaction

(70) Effective communication requires that a message have the strongest impact the ________ time it's communicated.

(A) First

(B) Second

(C) Tenth

(D) None of the above

(71) Which characteristic is considered unnecessary for building an effective relationship?

(A) Good communication

(B) Monitoring expenditures

(C) Sincere listening

(D) Positive presence as a leader

(72) The following are the five fundamental functions of ___________.

5. Making a plan.
6. Organizing resources and determining how to go about the changes.
7. Implementing the changes and making any necessary adjustments along the way.
8. Assessing the impact of the changes on a continued basis.
9. Seeking feedback.

(A) Budget management

(B) Financial planning

(C) Payment bundling

(D) Change management

(73) _______________ is/are defined as the money used to procure the inventory necessary to run an institution successfully.

(A) Revenue cycles

(B) Billable services

(C) Payment bundling

(D) Supply expenditures

(74) Which of the following is false regarding Just-in-time ordering?

(A) JIT ordering helps you avoid bidding for larger shipments

(B) JIT allows you to avoid having excess inventory

(C) JIT reduces inventory holding cost

(D) JIT increases inventory turnover

(75) Hospital XYZ spent $55,000 in 2021 and earned a profit of $33,650. Calculate the ROI hospital XYZ made during the year.

(A) 2.3%

(B) 1.5%

(C) 1.6%

(D) 2.2%

(76) ______________ is calculated by the money invested by the institution divided by the total number of hours worked. It provides an estimate of the institution's performance.

(A) Expenditure on labor

(B) Productivity

(C) ROI

(D) Depreciation

(77) An institution's productivity can be determined by all of the following except ________.

(A) Substitution

(B) Marginal productivity

(C) Expenditure on labor

(D) The short- and long-run

(78) __________ is the reimbursement method for health care services where the patient has to pay a particular payment called capitation.

(A) Point-of-service organization (POS)

(B) Medicare

(C) Health maintenance organizations (HMOs)

(D) Prospective payment system (PPS)

(79) What are the two binary scores on which the value-based purchasing program's scoring is based?

(A) 0 and 1

(B) Approved and disapproved

(C) 0 and 20

(D) 0 and 9

(80) Which of the following is not considered necessary when determining which vendor to purchase a product from?

(A) Terms and conditions of purchase

(B) A request for proposal

(C) The institution's financial plan

(D) How compatible the product is with the current equipment or software being used

(81) Group purchasing organizations (GPOs) are employed by many hospitals for ______.

(A) Sourcing material

(B) Productivity assessments

(C) Choosing a vendor

(D) Staff contract

(82) What type of employees should not be included in determining full-time equivalent (FTE)?

(A) Housekeeping employees

(B) Nursing staff

(C) Contractual employees

(D) Seasonal employees

(83) Revenue, expenses and statistics are the three primary features of a/an ________.

(A) Capital budget

(B) Cash budget

(C) Operating budget

(D) Master budget

(84) What is the 1947 Privacy Act?

(A) A law stating that the government has access to all and any information.

(B) A law restricting employee information that can be gathered and stored.

(C) A law stating that the personal information of patients can be handed out to anyone who asks for any reason.

(D) None of the above.

(85) How many steps are in Chally and Loriz's decision-making model?

(A) Four

(B) Eight

(C) Six

(D) Fifteen

(86) When was the decision-making model by Chally and Loriz introduced?

(A) 1965

(B) 1988

(C) 1998

(D) 2002

(87) How many provisions does the code of ethics for nurses have?

(A) Two

(B) Five

(C) Seven

(D) Nine

(88) Which of the following is not part of the code of ethics for nurses?

(A) Nurses are required to treat everyone with respect and consideration regardless of their social standing.

(B) Nurses have to tend to patients with total commitment, with all conflicts put aside.

(C) Nurses must uphold the privacy and confidentiality of a patient.

(D) Nurses can deny service to any patient asking for help.

(89) Which of the following is a fundamental right of all patients?

(A) To discriminate against nurses due to their social standing or a personal grudge

(B) To be respected by all medical staff, get a response when needed and decide what kind of medical care they'd like to receive

(C) To leave the hospital without paying any fees if they are unsatisfied with the treatment

(D) All of the above

(90) What does NCSBN stand for?

(A) The National Council of State Boards of Nursing

(B) The National Consultants of State Boards Nursing

(C) The National Consultants of State Board Nursing

(D) None of the above

(91) What is the NCSBN Model Act?

(A) A law that states all company information can be given out to any person who asks.

(B) A law that provides the model or outline that nursing boards should follow.

(C) A law that explains why technology integration is essential in medical care.

(D) None of the above.

(92) Which of the following is not a role of the Health Insurance Portability and Accountability Act (HIPAA)?

(A) Ensuring the privacy of patients' health status and their choice to keep it private

(B) Asking patients for consent before giving out their medical information to anyone

(C) Sharing the personal information of outpatients without regard for their safety

(D) Considering any current or past conditions or treatments patients have gone through as protected information that can't be given out

(93) What does the Genetic Information Nondiscrimination Act state?

(A) It states employers cannot decide whether or not to hire an individual based on genetics.

(B) It states employers can decide not to hire a person because of personal prejudice and dislike for the individual.

(C) It states employers can use individuals' genetics and personal race as reasons not to hire them.

(D) None of the above.

(94) Which of the following should not be included in emergency plans?

(A) Keeping any emergency supplies and necessities on hand at all times.

(B) Allowing and encouraging the staff to have access to any information on what to do in case of disasters or drills.

(C) Establishing a chain of command.

(D) Letting anyone willing to take leadership and command people.

(95) What is malpractice?

(A) Advising patients on the proper medical treatment or route best suited for them

(B) Any improper, illegal or negligent behavior in professional work, especially toward a client or patient

(C) A person who speaks up about fraudulent or wrongful activities in the workplace to a supervisor or anyone else internally to address the issue

(D) An employee who accuses innocent employees of committing fraudulent activities in the workplace to a supervisor or person of authority

(96) Which of the following is a form of negligent conduct?

(A) Tending to patients regardless of their social standing

(B) Failure to assist when asked to for no particular reason

(C) Giving total commitment to patients and tending to their medical needs

(D) Looking for medical solutions and advising patients to the best of your ability

(97) Who is a whistleblower?

(A) A person who speaks up about fraudulent or wrongful activities in the workplace to the supervisor or anyone else internally to address the issue

(B) An employee who commits fraudulent and wrongful acts in the workplace for their gain and benefit

(C) An employee who notices fraudulent behavior in the workplace but keeps quiet to stay out of trouble

(D) An employee who accuses innocent employees of committing fraudulent activities in the workplace to a supervisor or person of authority

(98) What is an example of unacceptable behavior when it comes to being professional?

(A) Doing the best that you can, but you fall short of the milestone you are trying to achieve

(B) Turning in a project past the deadline

(C) Not being punctual

(D) None of the above

(99) What is not a method of technological integration?

(A) Transmitting data of patients' blood pressure and heart rate using technology

(B) Interviewing patients through video calls

(C) Using phone calls to book appointments

(D) None of the above

(100) What is predictive analytics?

(A) Programs used by computers to find out about the needs of a health care organization by using existing data to predict the demands of patients 100 days in advance

(B) Services offered to people as outpatients, giving them access to physician offices, clinics, urgent care centers, surgery centers or hospitals

(C) Services for people who can't leave their homes, enabling the person who provides the service to travel to the patient's home

(D) Allowing the nurse assigned to monitor the patient through cameras or a screen without having to be in the same location

(101) Which of the following does not help with managing patient experience?

(A) Refusing patients based on personal preference or discrimination

(B) Letting employees commit an illegal act for their benefit or gain

(C) Not allowing patients to have a say in their treatment process

(D) All of the above

(102) Which of the following is not a factor used for health care delivery outcome evaluation?

(A) Health care consortium

(B) Leapfrog

(C) IHI bundles

(D) Healthgrade

(103) Which of the following is true about remote monitoring?

(A) It involves monitoring a patient through a screen or camera while the nurse is in another location physically.

(B) It involves being present in the same room when taking care of a patient.

(C) It involves more than two nurses watching over a patient.

(D) None of the above.

(104) When should an individual affected by a HIPAA breach be notified?

(A) One week

(B) Thirty days

(C) Sixty days

(D) Four months

(105) If the number of people affected by a HIPAA breach is around 10 or more, how long does the institution's website have to post information about the breach?

(A) One week

(B) One month

(C) Two months

(D) Three months

(106) Which act falls under ARRA and requires notifications be sent to individuals and the HHS in regard to security breaches of any information about a person's health?

(A) The Privacy Act of 1947

(B) The Nurse Practice Act

(C) The Health Information Technology for Economic and Clinical Health Act

(D) The NCSBN Model Act

(107) Which of the following falls under the categories of ACOs?

(A) Advanced payment model

(B) Pioneer model

(C) Shared savings program

(D) All of the above

(108) Which facilities provide a variety of services for the health improvements of their clients, including services not limited to medical care, such as feeding, bathing, etc.?

(A) Rehabilitation facilities

(B) Skilled nursing facilities

(C) Therapeutical facilities

(D) None of the above

(109) Which of the following are home-based care providers?

(A) Residential care facilities

(B) Assisted living facilities

(C) Facilities offering respite care

(D) All of the above

(110) A body charged with establishing the accreditation standards for single-person health care delivery programs is known as the ________.

(A) NSRA

(B) Single commission

(C) Double commission

(D) Joint commission

(111) Which insurance covers minor treatments, nursing and other health services at home, as well as hospital services for those with terminal illnesses?

(A) Medicare A insurance

(B) Medicare B insurance

(C) Healthgrade insurance

(D) Ambulatory insurance

(112) Health care services for outpatients are referred to as ________.

(A) Rehabilitation

(B) Pro bono

(C) Temporary services

(D) Ambulatory

(113) What is the following formula used to calculate?

(# of inpatient service days for period A ÷ # of bed-count days for inpatient during period A) x 100

(A) Rate of patients in the hospital

(B) Bed occupancy rate of inpatients

(C) Percentage of inpatients left

(D) None of the above

(114) What best defines the term “harassment”?

(A) Holding a grudge against a patient

(B) Refusing to tend to a patient because of personal reasons

(C) Making verbal utterances or physical contact that’s not welcomed by the other person

(D) Performing illegal actions

(115) What is an example of a platform that allows nurses to lobby for useful policies and the advancement of nursing as a profession?

(A) The National Nurse Board of Medicare

(B) The National Nursing Board of Medicare

(C) The American Organization of Nurse Executives

(D) None of the above

(116) What is an example of malpractice?

(A) Failing to refer a patient for treatment that may be necessary

(B) Giving the wrong diagnosis

(C) Not providing a guardian or family member with the necessary information

(D) All of the above

(117) Which of the following is a privately owned company that collects data of millions of health care providers and ranks them in terms of patient mortality and complication rates?

(A) Medicaid

(B) Healthgrade

(C) Leapfrog

(D) Health care

(118) Being compliant and adhering to state and federal laws is known as ________.

(A) Legality

(B) Abiding laws

(C) Cooperation

(D) Corporate compliance

(119) If a nurse purposefully disregards a patient's care or does not consider the person's safety, this falls under which of the following categories?

(A) Fraud

(B) Racism

(C) Discrimination

(D) Negligence

(120) A principle that requires health care providers not to do anything that may harm the patient is known as the ________.

(A) Principle of no maleficence

(B) Principle of maleficence

(C) Principle of nondiscrimination

(D) None of the above

(121) The act of misrepresenting information for personal gain or benefit is known as ______.

(A) Negligence

(B) Abandonment

(C) Malfunction

(D) Fraud

(122) For a clinic to be led by nurses, who must be in charge?

(A) A learning nurse

(B) A new nurse

(C) An advanced practice nurse

(D) An intern

(123) What is a program meant for the welfare of individuals that is managed by the federal and state government?

(A) Rehabilitation

(B) Healthgrade

(C) Medicaid

(D) Medicare A

(124) IHI bundles, ORYX ® indicators and Leapfrog are all examples of:

(A) Factors of health care delivery outcome evaluations

(B) Codes of ethics

(C) Company names

(D) All of the above

(125) Which of the following covers the costs of doctors, CNSs, lab tests, physical therapy and occupational therapy?

(A) Healthgrade

(B) Medicare B

(C) Medicare A

(D) Medicaid

(126) What is the primary role nurse executives play in an organization?

(A) They shape hospital policies within an organization.

(B) They provide nursing care to patients.

(C) They act as administrators overseeing the nursing program.

(D) They provide any health care that patients require.

(127) Which law protects the equal right to employment of disabled Americans?

(A) The Family and Medical Leave Act

(B) The National Labor Relations Act

(C) The Fair Labor Standards Act

(D) The American Disability Act

(128) Which of the following is not true about the FMLA?

(A) According to the FMLA, an employee can take a leave of around six weeks within a year.

(B) Acceptable conditions for an employee to qualify for unpaid leave under FMLA are either a medical issue or a family matter.

(C) An employee must work full or part time to qualify for an unpaid absence.

(D) According to the FMLA, the required time an employee should have served to qualify for an unpaid absence is 1250 hours in the previous year.

(129) Which wage and hour law protects employees from being exposed to unsanitary and unsafe working conditions?

(A) The Davis-Bacon Act

(B) The Walsh-Healey Public Contracts Act

(C) The Contract Work Hours & Safety Standards Act

(D) The Federal Wage Garnishment Law

(130) The Equal Employment Opportunity Commission (EEOC) oversees all the following organizations except for a/an ________.

(A) Small business of five employees

(B) Organization that ensures labor rights

(C) Employment agency

(D) Factory that has over 120 employees

(131) Which equal employment law protects employees against discrimination based on racial bias?

(A) The 1991 Civil Rights Act

(B) The 1967 ADEA

(C) The 1964 Civil Rights Act, Title VII

(D) The 1963 Equal Pay Act

(132) ________________________ is an organization that works toward making policies that help eliminate the risk of employees being exposed to infections.

(A) The Occupational Safety & Health Administration (OSHA)

(B) The Equal Employment Opportunity Commission (EEOC)

(C) The Walsh-Healey Public Contracts Act

(D) The Family & Medical Leave Act (FMLA)

(133) OSHA ensures that hospitals and health care organizations __________.

(A) Have a plan in place to reduce the risk of employee injury

(B) Adhere to universal precautionary measures

(C) Use modern technologies as they are introduced into the market

(D) Provide their staff with unpaid leave for 12 weeks a year

(134) What is not included in workers' compensation benefits?

(A) Monetary compensation as a substitute for lost wages due to recovery from sickness or injury

(B) Reimbursement for any expenses to treat the injury

(C) Days off are included and written off as unpaid absences

(D) The next of kin is paid any benefits received for the injured employee's death

(135) How can nurse executives benefit from knowledge of workers' compensation benefits?

(A) They can design appropriate and effective safety measures to minimize the risk of injury and illness.

(B) They can help avoid paying staff compensation benefits.

(C) They can realize the severity of the situation.

(D) They can garnish staff wages if they incur any onsite injuries.

(136) What is a reason employees can still sue their employer after receiving workers' compensation benefits?

(A) Garnishing wages as per the limit

(B) Reckless conduct

(C) Injury due to employee's carelessness

(D) Mental stress caused due to working overtime

(137) Which of the following does not comply with the Nursing Home Reform Amendments (NHRA) of 1990?

(A) The patients should be treated as per the Medicaid they use.

(B) A rehabilitation nurse can work only one shift a day.

(C) Patients should be assessed both mentally and physically upon admission.

(D) The state should maintain a registry of all the rehabilitation nurses working in its rehabilitation centers.

(138) Which of the following is not included in the 1965 Older Americans Act (OAA)?

(A) The provision of meals and transportation

(B) Protection from elder abuse

(C) The right to equal pay

(D) Services of a legal nature

(139) _____________ is a program through which OAA ensures that nursing homes are providing quality services to their elderly patients.

(A) The Omnibus Budget Reconciliation Act

(B) The Ombudsman

(C) The Nursing Home Reform Amendments of 1990

(D) The Family & Medical Leave Act

(140) Which law specifically addresses the need to provide high-quality health care services to any patient that comes into an ER, regardless of financial, racial, gender or religious background?

(A) The Occupational Safety & Health Administration

(B) The Emergency Medical Treatment & Active Labor Act

(C) The Family & Medical Leave Act

(D) The 1991 Civil Rights Act

(141) According to the EMTALA, which of the following is not a condition that needs to be satisfied for a patient to be transferred from the ER to a ward or another hospital?

(A) If the patient was in active labor, she should have delivered the baby and placenta.

(B) The patient's condition needs to be stable.

(C) The patient should be able to afford the hospital or ward charges.

(D) The health care provider needs to be confident that the patient's condition will not worsen due to the transfer.

(142) A delegation of nurses intends to approach the administration regarding their growing concerns about the unhygienic conditions in which the hospital cafeteria cooks the staff's lunch.

Which bargaining type is best suited to the task?

(A) Distributive negotiation

(B) Integrative negotiation

(C) Mixed negotiation

(D) None of the above

(143) Which of the following should not be factored in when negotiating contracts?

(A) The emotions of the concerned party

(B) Relevant data collection

(C) The expectations of the concerned party

(D) Notes and reports of recent negotiations

(144) If a dispute remains unresolved even after following the appropriate chain of command, then ______________ should be involved.

(A) A supervisor

(B) An arbitrator

(C) The union

(D) The immediate authority

(145) The following are the ___________________ a nurse executive should have excellent command over.

- Reflective communication
- Two-way communication
- The loop of feedback between the sender and receiver
- Hiring interview and motivational interviewing

(A) Labor issues

(B) Principles of communication

(C) Human resources

(D) Administrative strategies

(146) Which of the following is not included in active listening?

(A) The body language of the person

(B) Nonverbal communication

(C) A monologue

(D) Empathy

(147) _______________ is a conversation where both the parties involved in the conversation have the opportunity to express their opinions and arguments equally.

(A) Reflective communication

(B) Two-way communication

(C) The sender-receiver feedback loop

(D) Active listening

(148) Which of the following refers to the process where the originator composes a message intended to convey either a fact or opinion?

(A) Feedback

(B) Encoding

(C) Transmitting

(D) Decoding

(149) Stella has spent the day tirelessly working on a project that's due tomorrow. While she was busy working, her mother called her down to dinner, but as she was too occupied with her work, her mother's call fell on deaf ears.

What influences Stella's ability to decode the message?

(A) Inference

(B) Physical factors

(C) Psychological factors

(D) Context

(150) Which of the following factors is not relevant to staff hiring interviews?

(A) An applicant's work history and educational background

(B) The job description

(C) The applicant's ethnicity

(D) The federal and state laws applicable to the job

Test 3: Answers and Explanations

(1) (D) The Family and Medical Leave Act.

The Family and Medical Leave Act was established in 1993 and specifies rules and regulations regarding unpaid absences in case of acceptable reasons. It also lists a special concession for service members.

(2) (A) Twelve weeks.

One of the conditions for unpaid absence in the Family and Medical Leave Act includes 12 weeks of leave annually. The leave is granted on acceptable reasons that include medical reasons and family matters.

(3) (C) Concurrent benefits extended to 26 weeks per year.

The Family and Medical Leave Act includes a special concession for service members that may be extended to 26 weeks to care for a child or service member.

(4) (A) Civil rights of Americans with any kind of mental disability are respected, and those individuals are given an equal chance of employment.

The Americans with Disabilities Act (ADA) ensures the civil rights of American citizens with a disability. They are given equal chances of employment and have to be treated with respect.

(5) (B) They make sure that the ADA stipulations are adhered to and, if they are not, make the necessary recommendations.

Nurse executives are expected to be well versed in ADA stipulations.

(6) (D) Overtime begins counting after 40 working hours every week. Calculations are done at one and a half times the standard rate.

According to the FLSA, the minimum wage is $7.25 per hour. The average working hours are 40 a week, and overtime wages are calculated at one and a half times the standard rate.

(7) (C) The state can have its minimum wage above the federal minimum. Employees are entitled to higher salaries if state and federal wage laws vary.

The FLSA says that different states do not have to comply with the federal minimum wage. However, in that instance, a higher minimum wage has to be paid to the employee.

(8) (B) Employees should be paid the minimum or better wage if the contract's worth is below $2,500.

Under the McNamara-O'Hara Service Contract Act, employees are liable to a better or minimum wage if a contract is worth below $2,500.

(9) (C) The 1964 Civil Rights Act, Title VII.

The Pregnancy Discrimination Act is used along with the 1964 Civil Rights Act, Title VII, to ensure that employers do not discriminate against employees on a social basis.

(10) (A) The 1967 ADEA.

The Age Discrimination in Employment Act (ADEA) protects the rights of employees older than 40 years of age.

(11) (B) Comply with state regulations, even if they're more stringent than the ones set by OSHA.

The job of a nurse executive is to follow state rules, even if they are stricter compared to those set by OSHA.

(12) (C) Increase in wages and promotion after the employee rejoins the organization.

Workers' compensation does not state that there will be an increase in compensation or a promotion for injured employees after they rejoin the organization.

(13) (C) Single shift.

The NHRA promotes examinations that must be performed annually for a patient's physical and medical conditions. It also includes taking care of a patient on a 24-hour basis and states that RNs should be on duty for a minimum of a single shift a day.

(14) (B) The transfer is possible only when patients have been stabilized. If a patient is in labor, the transfer is only allowed when she has delivered both the baby and the placenta.

Transfer of patients can only be done when patients have been stabilized or delivered of both the baby and placenta. The receiving institution should have all the required facilities to treat the patients.

(15) (A) Matters revolving around wages and workplace conditions.

The CBA helps employees bargain collectively through their respective unions. The matters discussed include wages and workplace conditions.

(16) (D) Composite negotiation.

The three major bargaining types for labor negotiations include distributive, integrative and mixed.

(17) (D) Integrative bargaining.

Integrative bargaining promotes collaboration and helps parties bargain as partners in a positive environment. It also encourages resolving any problems and reaching a mutual decision.

(18) (B) Ensure that the negotiations are factual and not emotional.

As a nurse executive, your job is to ensure that contract negotiations are objective and only based on facts.

(19) (C) The cost of arbitration is split between both parties.

The immediate supervisor or any other authoritative entity has nothing to do with the cost of arbitration. Thus, it has to be divided between both parties.

(20) (B) Forty.

The NLRB facilitates a settlement to resolve disputes between employers and employees. The board has 40 judges that work with the NLRB to resolve the issues.

(21) (C) "I was saddened to hear of your loss. My staff and I send our condolences."

Empathy is crucial in active listening. You have to indicate that you comprehend what the other person is feeling and show that you genuinely care for their situation.

(22) (D) Vertical.

Two-way communication ensures that both parties are equally voicing their opinions. When a senior and someone junior interact, their two-way communication is described as vertical or downward.

(23) (A) It is the only way the encoder will know that the transmitted message has been received with its intended meaning.

The decoder has to provide feedback so that the encoder will know the message transmitted had the intended meaning.

(24) (B) "What is your ethnicity?"

The questions asked during an interview should only revolve around the job advertised. Asking any personal questions, such as about the employee's ethnicity or anything discriminatory, is not allowed.

(25) (C) Assertive.

An assertive form of communication shows somebody who has a calm, measured and positive tone. One way to recognize assertive communication is by using "I" statements.

(26) (B) Conflict.

Passive communication helps individuals communicate indirectly. In the short term, it helps avoid conflict.

(27) (B) Cross-training.

Cross-training enables staff members to handle different situations in the workplace. Proficiency in different tasks is essential, especially when staff members are rotated frequently.

(28) (C) It ensures that all staff positions are filled daily, even if someone is on leave.

Nurses use the accordion schedule to ensure no positions are left empty, even if a staff member is missing.

(29) (A) Age of the applicant.

The applicant's age should not be a factor when deciding on the best salary.

(30) (A) Three to five goals expected by the end of a given period and a success measuring rate.

The development of a plan of performance is the first step in employee performance management, and it focuses on outlining three to five goals with the target employee(s). The outcomes expected by the end of a given period should also be decided.

(31) (C) Focusing on streamlining your system instead of changing your employees' behavior.

A just culture promotes a focus on organizing a system instead of trying to change the individual's behavior. In that sense, it encompasses three major features: human error, risk behavior and reckless behavior.

(32) (C) Productive meetings between the employee and employer.

The matters important to the need for transparency in the workplace include disclosure of information, communication of information with accuracy and clarity in disseminating information.

(33) (D) The chief executive officer.

The command chain hierarchy has the institution governing body at the top, followed by the chief executive officer, then the nurse executive, the senior managers and so on.

(34) (C) Bottom-up structure.

Organizational charts depict the command chain pictorially. They also help demonstrate the relationship between different entities.

A hierarchical structure means that the chart follows a top-down structure. Other formats of organizational charts include matrix, horizontal and committee structure.

(35) (C) Has complex tasks and varies in nature.

The control span (the number of people being supervised) has to be defined when the organization has a hierarchical command chain.

When the work being performed has a routine nature, it is known as a *wide control span* since there are not a lot of instructions or directions to give.

In contrast, the *control span* is narrow when the work being performed has complex tasks and varies in nature.

(36) (B) Organization's size, nature of skills of employees, culture in the organization built over time, the nature of training supervisors have received and the responsibilities of different supervisors.

The optimal way to determine the best size of a control span includes taking the organization's size into account, along with the nature of skills the employees have. It also considers the nature of training supervisors have received, various supervisors' responsibilities and the organizational culture built over time.

(37) (A) Procedures explain the "why" of something, whereas policies talk about the "how" of something.

Policies and procedures both have clear instructions and use language that is easy to understand.

Policies explain the "why" behind an institution's mission statement, whereas procedures explain the "how" behind the mission statement. So, procedures are detailed when compared to policies.

(38) (D) Negotiation, communication, collaboration and conflict management.

Team performance management has four elements: negotiation, communication, collaboration and conflict management. Nurse executives must be fluent in each of these elements and should know how to deal with them in different settings.

(39) (C) Groups of form are homogenous in nature and have specific members that are only part of those groups.

Groups have the purpose of communication. For instance, groups of form are homogenous and have members specifically selected for them. An example of a group of form includes the staff of the OPD department. The staff members of this group stay within the group.

(40) (C) Emotions.

Emotions have no real contribution to bringing about any change. Effective change requires an individual to know why the change is being implemented.

The individual's knowledge about the change and the outcome it will bring about should be backed by the desire to make that change a reality. Whether or not the desired changes occur is backed by the individual's ability and the reinforcements behind it.

The acronym ADKAR was created to highlight the different steps an individual must take to bring about effective change.

(41) (C) They should have the relevant knowledge and skills to carry out the tasks to bring about the change.

Any people in charge of change management should have the relevant knowledge and skills to carry out the required tasks to bring about the needed change. If they don't, they won't be able to improve organizational culture and processes.

(42) (D) The six distinct phases that planned change undergoes.

It is necessary for nurse executives to understand how change comes about and the different steps it undergoes. This information can help them manage change more effectively.

Awareness, a desire to bring change, knowledge, ability and reinforcement (ADKAR) are integral to bringing about change on an individual level.

On an organizational or administrative level, the information must be systematically arranged so that administrators, such as nurse executives, can utilize it in change management.

(43) (A) Change management.

To promote a safety culture, an organization needs to promote accountability and risk management. One method of implementing a safety culture is providing the necessary gear for the staff to practice their skills safely.

The staff needs to be made aware of why they must follow the steps put in place to reduce the risk of any potential danger to them or the patients.

(44) (C) Risks can be desired.

Risks are uncertain circumstances that can potentially lead to negative results. However, they can be managed by identifying factors that can prove to be risks and then mitigating them.

(45) (C) Being well-versed in federal and state laws.

Effective leadership requires an administrator to create an environment that promotes a sense of safety and empowerment. Such an environment will provide the staff with the circumstances that can help them achieve total customer satisfaction or, as in the case of health care organizations, patient satisfaction.

(46) (C) An institution with policies in place to prevent bullying and other forms of violence.

A safe environment is essential for an institution to function optimally. The institution should provide its employees with adequate training and awareness to ensure their safety and the safety of the patients they look after.

The institution should also have fire escapes and alarms in case of an emergency. Good lighting and air quality are crucial for the institution's employees and patients who come there to receive health care services.

An institution that does nothing to prevent bullying and other forms of violence in its environment can never function properly.

(47) (D) Allow employees a certain level of autonomy per their respective positions.

Staff empowerment requires the administration to train and make staff aware of the information necessary to perform their duties.

Good leadership does not micromanage employees; instead, it allows them to work with the level of independence their positions require. Reducing discrimination against employees or wage garnishment can contribute to staff satisfaction.

On the other hand, an administration's expectation of punctuality from employees is an essential requirement that needs to be fulfilled for the organization to operate normally.

(48) (A) Flexible work schedule.

Allowing employees to have flexible work hours can increase staff satisfaction. The administration should consider providing employees with a positive environment to work in, free of unjust garnishing of wages and discrimination.

(49) (A) The Plan-Do-Check-Act Cycle.

The PDCA Cycle, also known as the Deming Cycle, is a repetitive cycle that teaches us how to manage, study and act upon our observations. Lean Six Sigma is a method used to improve processes in a manufacturing environment.

Root cause analysis is a preventive measure that resolves issues by eliminating and mitigating different sources of the issue. It does not attempt to resolve issues by remedying their symptoms.

(50) (A) Lean Six Sigma.

The method for process improvement utilized in manufacturing environments is known as Lean Six Sigma. It is a six-step method that comprises:

- Recognize
- Define
- Measure
- Analyze
- Improve
- Cycle.

The repetitive cycle used by nurses to help manage employees, data and risks is called the PDCA cycle. It demonstrates the importance of observation and how to use the information acquired from it when managing things.

A root cause analysis allows nurse executives to resolve issues from the very source rather than finding a temporary fix for the issue's symptoms.

(51) (C) Knowledge management.

Methods used to continuously improve on different processes that run an organization and research allow nurse executives to manage knowledge. Knowledge management enables them to perform their administrative duties more effectively.

(52) (D) Root cause analysis.

A root cause analysis is considered preventative in its methodology of resolving issues as it aims to eradicate a problem at its core.

Other continuous process improvement methods, such as the PDCA Cycle and Lean Six Sigma, are more focused on treating the symptoms of the issue.

(53) (B) They should be conversant with the laws put in place by the Institutional Review Board (IRB) and FDA.

To protect people who agree to become research subjects, nurse executives need to be well-versed in the laws created to protect such individuals. They should also know the different boards, such as the IRB, FDA and HHI, created to oversee research subject protection.

(54) (D) Performance enhancement.

Nurse executives who possess research knowledge can utilize it to improve their administrative methodology, helping them enhance the overall performance of their organization.

(55) (C) Protecting research subjects.

To successfully advocate a positive environment that promotes research, a nurse executive can bring about different initiatives, like creating journal clubs where professionals can come together and review scientific journals and relevant literature that can help them improve the institution's overall performance.

They can also apply for grants to receive funding that can help the researchers in their institutes effectively conduct their studies.

(56) (A) They can help implement modern technologies and techniques.

Knowledge management is possible by studying innovation as it allows individuals to learn how to implement innovative techniques and how to use innovative equipment.

It also enables them to successfully incorporate respective innovations anywhere they can to improve their organization's administration and overall performance.

(57) (C) To ensure patients' health and safety.

Systems theory in nursing refers to possessing the knowledge necessary to create a health care system that ensures patient safety and health are prioritized. The theory is turned into practices that work toward making the entire health care system more efficient.

(58) (B) Innovation management theory.

Organic systems have conditions liable to change, whereas mechanical systems are more stabilized. Innovation management theory compares systems to study their unique culture, context and product.

(59) (C) Organic.

An organic system is subject to more changes than a mechanical system because it has low centralization, complexity and formalization. So, any change in these conditions can bring about a substantial effect.

(60) (C) Innovations.

Innovation is not included in the five distinct disciplines of a learning institution. These principles are based on how to bring about favorable changes that help further the continuous transformation of learning organizations.

(61) (B) System thinking.

Systems thinking is a holistic approach that views an organization as a whole. It observes and analyzes the departments and units that compose an organization and studies their interrelated work.

(62) (C) The staff.

The continuous quality improvement (CQI) theory focuses more on an institution's structure. It analyzes the different components of the structure and views the employees working within the organization as internal customers and patients as external customers.

(63) (A) FOCUS.

The performance enhancement model that facilitates change within an organization is called FOCUS. It is an acronym for *find, organize, clarify, uncover* and *start*. These are the systematic steps of the entire process:

- *Find:* Any issues the organization faces are identified.
- *Organize:* A team skilled enough to resolve the problem is brought together.
- *Clarify:* Team members brainstorm potential solutions for a problem.
- *Uncover*: Team members try to uncover the underlying cause of the issue.
- *Start*: The solution begins to be implemented.

(64) (B) Clarify.

FOCUS is a performance model with different steps to identify organizational problems. The step where other skilled team members brainstorm to come up with a potential solution to the problem is *clarify*.

(65) (B) Employee empowerment.

A clinical outcome refers to the quantitative and qualitative changes in a patient's health that are a direct outcome of health care provided by an organization. It does not involve employee empowerment.

(66) (C) A year.

A financial plan is defined as a framework of a business's finances and growth trajectory. The information a financial plan strategizes to record cannot be curated over the short duration of a month. However, durations of five years and a decade are both too long to wait to apply the findings realized from the analysis of financial activities.

An organization can develop long- or short-term financial plans. But generally, a year is considered the best time frame to acquire the necessary information to develop a business strategy based on facts and figures that result from how successful your long- and short-term business goals have been.

(67) (B) Budget management.

Budgeting is when an estimated amount of money is allocated for particular tasks at the beginning of the year, e.g., when money is set aside for variable or petty cash costs.

Effective budgeting can help a business or organization achieve its financial goals. It also helps track the total incoming revenue and the expenditures made during the financial year. Plus, it ensures that the goals for the financial year are met.

In contrast, expenditure control is essentially monitoring the resources of the organization and how they are being spent. It ensures whether or not the limitations set in the budget management are being followed.

The evaluation of costs incurred is another option that's retrospective and enables feedback on financial performance.

(68) (D) Payer system.

A payer system is a reimbursement method for health care services an organization provides. It includes a variety of methods by which a patient can pay for the services provided by the health care organization.

These methods include self-pay, health maintenance organizations (HMOs), prospective payment systems (PPS), preferred provider organizations (PPOs), point-of-service organizations (POSs) and Medicare.

In contrast, a revenue cycle is a series of categorical steps by which billing is done in an organization. The components of a revenue cycle are:

1. Registration or preregistration

2. Billable services

3. Coding

4. Chargemaster

5. Capture

6. Submission

7. Resubmission or appeals

8. Collection.

(69) (B) Effective communication.

Nurse executives must master verbal and nonverbal communication skills to ensure an effective relationship with their staff and patients.

When communicating, they should be able to read any message communicated symbolically. They should also be able to communicate in symbolic language effectively.

(70) (A) First.

Communication depends on the receiver's understanding and perception. To effectively communicate, it's best to remember to use the tone, style and language suited to conveying the intended message to the receiver.

How the message is first communicated has the strongest effect due to its impact on the receiver. For example, if nurse executives do not take into account the need to communicate the severity of a patient's condition in the correct tone and manner, they run the risk of offending the patient, which can cause more mental and physical suffering.

So, communication should be viewed as a skill that needs to be assessed with the receiver's context in mind.

(71) (B) Monitoring expenditures.

To build effective relationships, nurse executives should prioritize the environment they create for those working around them. Good leaders encourage good communication and sincere listening. They do not monitor expenditures.

(72) (D) Change management.

Any business can be subject to changes that might disrupt normal day-to-day operations. The nurse executive is responsible for managing such changes in a manner that keeps the institution functioning smoothly.

(73) (D) Supply expenditures.

The money spent by an organization to acquire the supplies needed to run its operations smoothly is called supply expenditure. It is utilized for materials or equipment as deemed necessary by the organization.

Revenue cycles are a series of categorical steps followed within an organization to process a patient's billing, while billable services are a part of the revenue cycle. They refer to the diagnostic services provided to the patient by the hospital.

Payment bundling is a method of reimbursing health care providers for the services provided to the patient rather than paying each provider separately.

(74) (A) JIT helps you avoid bidding for larger shipments.

Most institutions have an automatic reordering system in place for their inventory. Just-in-time ordering minimizes the cost of holding large inventory, helps keep expenditures under budget and leads to less time spent in ordering the ordered supplies in small quantities.

(75) (C) 1.6%.

Return on investment (ROI) is a measurement of the profit earned by an institution on an initial investment. It is given as a percentage and is calculated by dividing the profit by the total investment and multiplying the resulting answer by a hundred.

The ROI for hospital XYZ would be: ($33,650÷ $55,000) x 100 = 1.6%.

(76) (B) Productivity.

As organizations like hospitals primarily provide health care services, their performance is determined by their productivity.

Productivity is quantified by measuring the ratio of output to input. It can also be measured by dividing the total amount of money invested by the total number of hours worked throughout a particular time period.

Expenditure on labor refers to an organization's expense for paying their employees overtime pay. ROI is the percentage of the profit made by an organization for the resources used over a particular time.

Depreciation is the amount of money that any fixed asset or equipment owned by the organization depreciates over time.

None of the other options are correct measures of whether or not an organization is performing optimally.

(77) (C) Expenditure on labor.

Expenditure on labor comes under the umbrella of budget management. It states the amount of money spent on staff for overtime, but it does not in any manner determine the overall productivity of the institution.

On the other hand, marginal productivity determines what an institute produces for every unit of resource spent by it, while short- and long-run entail the time spent per activity by an institute.

Substitution refers to replacing costly input with a more inexpensive one. These three terms refer to data contributing to the institute's overall productivity.

(78) (C) Health maintenance organizations (HMOs).

HMOs are a type of payer system that allows a patient to pay a set amount for an overall service package. This set fee is called capitation.

(79) (D) 0 and 9.

Value-based purchasing is an incentivized rewards system created by CMS to ensure quality health care. The assessment is based on whether or not the health care provided is above the set threshold.

If the hospital scores above the threshold, it's given a score of 9. If it is below the threshold, it's given a score of 0.

(80) (C) The institution's financial plan.

When considering which vendor to use to supply the material your institute requires, it is crucial to research their services and product. This includes the product history, how compatible it is with your current equipment and software and whether or not it has any updates.

Other factors you need to consider are the terms and conditions of the purchase, whether or not the vendor is willing to provide the required services to help train your staff, and maintenance.

(81) (A) Sourcing material.

Institutions like hospitals employ group purchasing organizations (GPOs) to simplify the process of sourcing the materials they need.

There are many benefits of sourcing material through GPOs, one of which is that as these organizations work for multiple institutions, they can easily acquire material in bulk for much cheaper.

Sourcing material through GPOs has been proven to help save on supply expenditures by 10 to 15%.

(82) (D) Seasonal employees.

Full-time equivalent (FTE) is a measurement of staff productivity based on their total hours worked during a period.

The official FTE hours are 2,080 hours for a year's worth of work hours. This is the standard for full-time employees. The work hours for seasonal employees are 120 hours a year.

As the total number of work hours of seasonal employees is not equal to the standardized FTE hours, seasonal employees are not included in determining FTE.

(83) (C) Operating budget.

The budget allocated for running the day-to-day operations of an institute is called an operating budget. It is determined by the revenue, expenses and statistics of particular operations. These operations may include employee salaries, depreciation, expenditure on labor and supply expenditure. The operating budget also consists of the profit generated through the above activities.

In contrast, a capital budget includes expenditures that address long-term needs, such as buying new equipment or renovations. These long-term needs are to be fulfilled within the year's budget.

The cash budget refers to the cash flow that the organization has throughout the year. It includes any money directly spent and received. A substantial cash budget ensures the organization has the required money for anticipated expenses.

The master budget is an umbrella term that includes all the items of operating, capital and cash budgets. It may also include any other budget an institution sets for a special reason other than those previously anticipated.

(84) (B) A law restricting employee information that can be gathered and stored.

The 1947 Privacy Act restricts the kinds of information that can be gathered and stored in someone's files. It provides direction for laws that are fair toward information practices collected, maintained and used, as well as distribution of such information about people and is upheld by a system of records by federal agencies.

(85) (C) Six.

The model's six steps show ethical ways to make wise decisions:

1. Clarify the problem/dilemma.
2. Gather any information needed.
3. Be aware of the options you have.
4. Make a decision.

5. Act on the decision.
6. Observe and evaluate the impact acting on the decision had.

(86) (C) 1998.

Chally and Loriz created their decision-making model in 1998.

(87) (D) Nine.

The nine provisions of the code of ethics of nurses are:

1. Treat everyone with respect and consideration regardless of their or your social standing.
2. Commit to a patient completely without letting conflicts get in the way.
3. Promote and tend to the health and safety of all patients.
4. Uphold a patient's privacy and confidentiality.
5. Take responsibility for all practices carried out.
6. Exercise self-respect, keep up integrity and be competent.
7. Contribute to the environment by aiding health care.
8. Develop any knowledge to advance in your profession as a nurse.
9. Collaborate and work with other medical staff to meet the patient's needs.

(88) (D) Nurses can deny service to any patient asking for help.

Nurses cannot deny service or refuse to tend to a patient without valid reasoning or for personal grudges and emotions, as it is against a nurse's code of ethics.

(89) (B) To be respected by all medical staff, get a response when needed and decide what kind of medical care they'd like to accept.

Patients have the right to be taken care of respectfully by medical staff and to decide the medical care they'd like to receive.

(90) (A) The National Council of State Boards of Nursing.

NCSBN stands for the National Council of State Boards of Nursing.

(91) (B) A law that provides the model or outline that nursing boards should follow.

The NCSBN acts as a model or outline for all nursing boards to follow.

(92) (C) Sharing the personal information of outpatients without regard for their safety.

A company is held accountable for any patients' personal information and is responsible for keeping it safe and away from anyone not authorized to see it.

(93) (A) It states employers cannot decide whether or not to hire an individual based on genetics.

The Genetic Information Nondiscrimination Act states that employers cannot make decisions on whether or not to hire an individual based on the person's genetics.

(94) (D) Letting anyone willing to take leadership and command people.

During an emergency, a proper chain of command should be established early on to keep people calm and avoid any confusion.

(95) (B) Any improper, illegal or negligent behavior in professional work, especially toward a client or patient.

Malpractice is any improper, illegal or negligent behavior in professional work, especially toward a client or patient.

(96) (B) Failure to assist when asked to for no particular reason.

Failing to assist a patient for no reason or personal reasons/emotions, such as prejudice or discrimination, falls under a form of malpractice known as negligence.

(97) (A) A person who speaks up about fraudulent or wrongful activities in the workplace to the supervisor or anyone else internally to address the issue.

A whistleblower is someone who speaks up about fraudulent or wrongful activities in the workplace to the supervisor or anyone else internally to address an issue.

(98) (C) Not being punctual.

Puntuality is important and a part of professionalism.

(99) (C) Using phone calls to book appointments.

Technological integration means using technology in everyday appliances in clinics and hospitals to make data storage and updates easier to keep track of.

A phone call has been a normal way of booking appointments for years. Technological integration means it'll be replaced by programs like Calendly in the future.

(100) (A) Programs used by computers to find out about the needs of a health care organization by using existing data to predict the demands of patients 100 days in advance.

A predictive analysis is performed by programs to find out about the needs of a health care organization by using existing data to predict the demands of patients more than 100 days in advance.

(101) (D) All of the above.

The steps to manage patient experiences are as follows:

1. Offer patients easier ways to schedule their appointments through the internet, phone or in person.
2. Act friendly and pay attention to their needs.
3. Have any forms they may need to fill out available online.
4. Ensure a clean and comfortable waiting room.
5. Respond to any feedback.
6. Keep in touch with patients.

(102) (D) Healthgrade.

The factors used for health care delivery outcome evaluations include:

1. Leapfrog
2. IHI bundles
3. ORYX® indicators
4. National patient safety goals
5. Health care buyer's consortium
6. Magnet recognition program.

(103) (A) It involves monitoring a patient through a screen or camera while the nurse is in another location physically.

Remote monitoring is a useful way to keep an eye on patients by observing them through a camera or screen in a different location. It is also helpful for monitoring quarantined patients.

(104) (C) Sixty days.

If an individual is affected, he or she should be notified within 60 days. However, if 10 or so individuals are affected, they should be notified through a website post in about three months, and if hundreds of individuals are affected, they must be notified through a public media alert.

(105) (D) Three months.

If 10 or so individuals are affected by a HIPAA breach, they must be notified through a website post in about three months.

(106) (C) The Health Information Technology for Economic and Clinical Health Act.

The Health Information Technology for Economic and Clinical Health Act falls under ARRA. It requires notifications to be sent to individuals and the HHS in regard to security breaches of any information about a person's health.

(107) (D) All of the above.

The different categories of ACO are shared savings, advance payment and pioneer model.

(108) (B) Skilled nursing facility.

Skilled nursing facilities provide a variety of services for their clients, including medical and personal care services, such as feeding, bathing, etc.

(109) (D) All of the above.

Residential care facilities, assisted-living facilities and facilities offering respite care are home-based care providers.

(110) (D) Joint commission.

A joint commission exists when someone is charged with establishing the accreditation standards for single-person health care delivery programs.

(111) (A) Medicare A insurance.

Medicare A is an insurance plan that covers minor treatments, nursing and other health services at home and in hospitals for those with terminal illnesses.

(112) (D) Ambulatory.

Ambulatory health care services are offered to people as outpatients rather than inpatients. These patients are usually treated in offices, clinics, urgent care centers, surgery centers or hospitals.

(113) (B) Bed occupancy rate of inpatients.

The formula calculates the bed occupancy rate of patients: (No. of inpatient service days for period A ÷No. of bed-count days (inpatient) for period A) x 100.

(114) (C) Making verbal utterances or physical contact that's not welcomed by the other person.

The term "harassment" is best defined as any verbal utterances or physical touching that are not welcomed by the other person and are being done without their mutual consent.

(115) (C) The American Organization of Nurse Executives.

The American Organization of Nursing Executives is one of the many platforms nurses use to lobby and petition for useful policies and the advancement of nursing as a profession.

(116) (D) All of the above.

Malpractice is any negligent, improper or illegal behavior expressed in a professional setting. Any unprofessional behavior and lack of providing a patient/client with the needs or services they pay for is considered malpractice.

(117) (B) Healthgrade.

Healthgrade is a privately owned company that collects data from millions of health care providers and ranks them in terms of patient mortality and complication rates.

(118) (D) Corporate compliance.

Corporate compliance is when companies and organizations adhere to every state and federal law.

(119) (D) Negligence.

Negligence occurs when someone fails to take proper care of something or someone. In this case, it may refer to the client or patient care.

(120) (A) Principle of no maleficence.

The principle of no maleficence states that health care providers must make sure they do not do anything that may harm patients.

(121) (D) Fraud.

Fraud is the act of misrepresenting information for personal gain or benefit. It is a malpractice category, and there are a few types of fraud in this case.

One case includes theft of medical identification, which happens when a person's medical identification number is misused by someone else so they can benefit from health care services or medical supplies. It may even be used to receive prescriptions illegally.

Fraud can also include billing unneeded items for the hospital.

(122) (C) An advanced practice nurse.

An advanced practice nurse must oversee a clinic run by nurses.

(123) (C) Medicaid.

Medicaid is a program designed specifically for the welfare of individuals and is managed by the federal and state government.

(124) (A) Factors of health care delivery outcome evaluations.

IHI bundles, ORYX ® indicators and Leapfrog are all factors and companies that evaluate health care delivery outcomes.

(125) (B) Medicare B.

Medicare B is an insurance policy covering the costs of doctors, CNSs, lab tests, physical therapy and occupational therapy.

(126) (C) They act as administrators overseeing the nursing program.

Nurse executives perform all the administrative duties in any hospital. Their role includes ensuring that the staff has everything required to provide patients with quality health care. They are also responsible for executing plans and policies to run an effective nursing program.

(127) (D) The Americans with Disabilities Act.

The Americans with Disabilities Act specifically protects the equal rights of employment of any disabled Americans. It includes people who are either mentally or physically impaired.

FMLA is a law that ensures any organization with a workforce of 50 or more provides part- or full-time employees with the right to unpaid absences.

FLSA is a policy that stipulates the standard minimum wage and the rate of overtime for employees. It also maintains laws for what is considered child labor.

NLRA looks after the collective rights of employees to protect them from companies that exploit their workers.

(128) (A) According to the FMLA, an employee can take a leave of around six weeks within a year.

The FMLA allows an employee that's either employed part- or full-time by the company 12 weeks of unpaid absence in the span of a year.

(129) (C) The Contract Work Hours & Safety Standards Act.

The Contract Work Hours & Safety Standards Act is the wage and hour law that prohibits employers from exposing their workers to unsanitary and unsafe working conditions.

The law also ensures that employees working on a project with a worth exceeding $100 or $1,000 in value are paid overtime at the rate of one and a half times per hour for every hour over 40 hours a week.

The Davis-Bacon Act is a law that ensures that contractors or subcontractors working on any public project are paid at the highest current rate in the market.

The Walsh-Healey Public Contracts Act establishes the set rate for minimum and overtime wages for any worker employed by the government for a project that exceeds $10,000 in value.

The Federal Wage Garnishment Law limits the extent to which an employee's wages can be garnished.

(130) (A) Small business of five employees.

The EEOC protects employees against discrimination. The organizations it monitors must have 15 or more employees. So, option A, a small business with five employees, is the exception.

The EEOC also monitors labor unions and employment agencies to ensure equal work opportunities for everyone.

(131) (C) The 1964 Civil Rights Act, Title VII.

The 1964 Civil Rights Act, Title VII, protects employees against discrimination based on their race. It also includes discrimination against gender, country of origin, religion and pregnancy.

In contrast, the 1991 Civil Rights Act specifically addresses the role of nurse executives. It refers to the amendments to the previous laws that address financial compensation and punitive damages.

Similarly, the 1963 Equal Pay Act states that employers should pay their employees equal wages as long as they perform the same work at the same quality. And the 1967 ADEA protects employees against discrimination against age. It mainly refers to employees who are aged 40 and above.

(132) (A) The Occupational Safety and Health Administration (OSHA).

OSHA is an organization working toward implementing policies that protect employees from infections.

In contrast, the EEOC ensures that employees are afforded equal employment rights and are not discriminated against or exploited.

The Walsh-Healey Public Contracts Act is a law that has set a standardized rate for minimum and overtime wages for employees working on government-funded projects valued at over $10,000.

On the other hand, FMLA is a law to ensure part- and full-time employees are afforded unpaid leaves without the threat of termination by their employers.

(133) (D) Provide their staff with unpaid leave for 12 weeks in a year.

OSHA's main objective is to ensure that health care employees work in safe environments. It does not monitor the medical staff's unpaid leaves or wages.

(134) (C) Days off are included and written off as unpaid absences.

Workers' compensation benefits include monetary compensation for any days off work an injured or sick employee has to incur. So, this leave is not unpaid.

Other benefits include reimbursement for any medical treatment a worker has to undergo due to an injury. If the employee passes away due to the injury or illness contracted in the line of duty, the next of kin will receive any benefits that were to be paid.

(135) (A) They can design appropriate and effective safety measures to minimize the risk of injury and illness.

Nurse executives act as administrators in the nursing program. The knowledge that comes from being well-informed about workers' compensation benefits can help them strategize and put into place policies that can prevent or reduce the risk of injury substantially. It can also enable them to design effective staff training sessions.

(136) (B) Reckless conduct.

If an employee suffers an injury while doing a job requiring special protection, which the employer failed to provide, then the employee can sue the employer for reckless conduct.

(137) (A) The patients should be treated as per the Medicaid they use.

According to the Nursing Home Reform Amendments (NHRA) of 1990, a patient should not be discriminated against on any basis, especially Medicaid. The amendments ensure that both the staff and patients in rehabilitation centers have policies that protect their well-being.

Patients must be assessed upon admission and annually, and rehabilitation nurses are provided with the necessary resources to perform their duties.

(138) (C) The right to equal pay.

The Older Americans Act ensures that Native Americans and elder citizens are provided enhanced services that allow them to lead better lives. These services include providing meals and transportation, home care, home repairs, services of a legal nature, protection against abuse and opportunities for computer literacy.

It does not, however, include the right to employment or the right to equal pay. The 1967 ADEA is a law that protects employees against discrimination against age.

(139) (B) The Ombudsman.

The Ombudsman is a program sanctioned by the OAA that provides elderly patients residing in nursing homes a platform to express their concerns or complaints. This allows the system to ensure that nursing homes are providing the standard of health care and rehabilitation services required by their respective states.

(140) (B) The Emergency Medical Treatment & Active Labor Act.

EMTALA was created to ensure that any patient who comes into an emergency room is provided with the required health care services, regardless of whether or not that individual can pay for them.

(141) (C) The patient should be able to afford the hospital or ward charges.

The primary concern that EMTALA addresses is that no patients are discriminated against in an ER based on whether or not they can afford medical treatment.

(142) (B) Integrative negotiation.

Integrative negotiation is a type of bargaining where both parties work toward a mutually agreed-upon solution. The given situation's problem is a concern for both parties, so an integrative negotiation is best suited to resolve the problem.

In contrast, distributive negotiation is a manner of bargaining where there is no room for compromise. It presents a win-or-lose situation. Mixed negotiation utilizes strategies from both integrative and distributive negotiations.

(143) (A) The emotions of the concerned party.

Nurse executives should ensure that negotiations are based on facts acquired from relevant data collection and previous negotiations. They should not be subject to the emotions of either of the concerned parties.

(144) (B) An arbitrator.

An arbitrator is an impartial third-party person with no stake in a dispute. The facts of the matter should be presented to the arbitrator. The concerned parties should adhere to the decision the arbitrator makes.

(145) (B) Principles of communication.

The given skills are the principles of communication that nurse executives need to adhere to manage their administrative role in any health care organization successfully.

(146) (C) A monologue.

A monologue occurs when a receiver is not actively participating in the conversation. Active listening requires the listener to attentively listen to what another person has to say and be emphatic in how they perceive it.

(147) (B) Two-way communication.

Two-way communication is a type of conversation where both participants have an equal opportunity to express their opinions, arguments and supporting facts.

(148) (B) Encoding.

Encoding is the step in the process of effective communication where the person intending to convey some form of information initially writes a message.

(149) (C) Psychological factors.

In the given situation, Stella's ability to decode her mother's message was impaired due to psychological factors. She was too busy with her work to decode her mother's message.

(150) (C) The applicant's ethnicity.

The person conducting the interview should assess whether or not the applicant is qualified for the job. The questions should be relevant in assessing their knowledge and skills.

Discriminatory questions related to age, gender, religion or race are not permissible during interviews.

Made in the USA
Middletown, DE
05 March 2023